Practical Skin Pathology

Diya F. Mutasim

Practical Skin Pathology

Springer

Diya F. Mutasim
Dept. of Dermatology and
Dermatopathology
University of Cincinnati College
of Medicine
Cincinnati
Ohio
USA

ISBN 978-3-319-14728-4 ISBN 978-3-319-14729-1 (eBook)
DOI 10.1007/978-3-319-14729-1

Library of Congress Control Number: 2015930839

Springer Cham Heidelberg New York Dordrecht London

Printed on acid-free paper

Springer is part of Springer Science+Business Media (www.springer.com)

To my sons Danny and Adam

Preface

Why This Book?

> "As is your pathology, so is your medicine,"
> William Osler

The father of modern American medicine acknowledged that a practitioner's medical practice is as good as their knowledge of pathology. It is with his spirit that this book was conceived and with his wisdom that its goals were identified.

As a dermatologist, a dermatopathologist, and a teacher of both disciplines, I have faced questions from residents and practitioners that have no straightforward answers in published textbooks of clinical dermatology and dermatopathology. This book was written to answer these questions and as a supplement to major textbooks on clinical and histological diagnosis of skin disorders.

The goal of this book is to help students of dermatology and practitioners cross the space between clinical dermatology and dermatopathology in order to improve their comprehension of skin disorders and further help manage their patients.

The book is divided into two parts.

The first part addresses histological diagnoses that do not have single and specific clinical counterparts, for example, psoriasiform dermatitis, lichenoid dermatitis, atypical melanocytic hyperplasia, pseudolymphoma, etc.

The second part addresses ways to use the clinical and histological findings to arrive at the best diagnosis in a patient presenting with:

- A certain lesion morphology, for example, eczematous, papulo-squamous, nodular, edematous, sclerotic, bullous, generalized pruritus, etc. and
- Lesions on specific sites of the body, such as scalp pustules, face papules, leg nodules, palmoplanter hyperkeratosis, patchy scalp alopecia, etc.

What This Book Does Not Claim to Accomplish

This is not a book teaching the histopathology of skin disorders. There are many such books that accomplish their goals brilliantly. The material here is not likely to prepare a resident for the board examination, or a practitioner for recertification.

Instead, this book aims to help the clinical practitioner learn about the power of histopathology but also its many limitations. Understanding the power and limitations would hopefully lead to more effective and more efficient practice and use of resources. It would also hopefully help practitioners ask for specific pathology answers to their clinical questions, accept limited answers to others, and learn how to tell the difference between the two situations.

The clinical and histological knowledge and opinion that is contained in this book is the result of 35 years of study, a long consultative clinical practice, and interpretation of hundreds of thousands of biopsy specimens in a university practice setting.

Practical Skin Pathology

As is your pathology, so is your medicine
William Osler, internist 1849–1919

A need existed for dermatohistology in order to understand fully the clinical facts
Josef Kyrle, dermatologist 1880–1926

Our responsibility is not to rest till we have brought the macro and microscopical appearances into agreement one with the other
Paul Gerson Unna, dermatologist and dermatopathologist 1850–1929

Pathology is not a pure science. The pathological changes are merely one side of a problem of which the other side is furnished by the clinical picture. Each throws light upon the other, and neither is complete by itself
William Boyd, pathologist 1885–1979

It is of the highest importance in the art of detection to be able to recognize out of a number of facts which are incidental and which vital
Arthur Conan Doyle, doctor and author 1859–1930

As no two faces, so no two cases are alike in all respects
William Osler, internist 1849–1919

First is the patient
Bela Schick, pediatrician 1877–1967

Contents

Part I
The pathologist's view

Chapter 1
What is Atypical Junctional Melanocytic Hyperplasia?

Figure 1.1 illustrates cases with disorders discussed in this chapter.

Junctional Melanocytic Hyperplasia

The term "junctional melanocytic hyperplasia" (JMH) refers to the proliferation of melanocytes along the dermo–epidermal junction that is the basal layer where normal melanocytes reside. JMH is not a clinical diagnosis but a histological term, just as epidermal hyperplasia or nodular lymphocytic infiltrate. JMH generally refers to the proliferation of single melanocytes rather than nests of melanocytes, and is characteristic of *lentigo simplex*; hence, the term *lentiginous* is often used to describe this finding.

Some pathologists make the diagnosis of *lentiginous nevus* for a junctional nevus with prominent lentiginous (or single cell) melanocytic hyperplasia. Others use the term *jentigo* to describe such proliferation, implying a lesion with features of both lentigo and early junctional nevus. Clinically, these lesions are usually very dark but small. Biologically, they represent the early stages of a melanocytic nevus and are common in childhood and youth. It is their dark and sometimes black color that causes concern by the patient, leading to their excision. Both, lentigo simplex and lentiginous junctional nevus are easily diagnosed histologically.

What Other Lesions May Reveal JMH?

As mentioned in the discussion on *dysplastic nevus*, JMH is a key histological feature in dysplastic nevi and melanoma.

D. F. Mutasim, *Practical Skin Pathology*, DOI 10.1007/978-3-319-14729-1_1

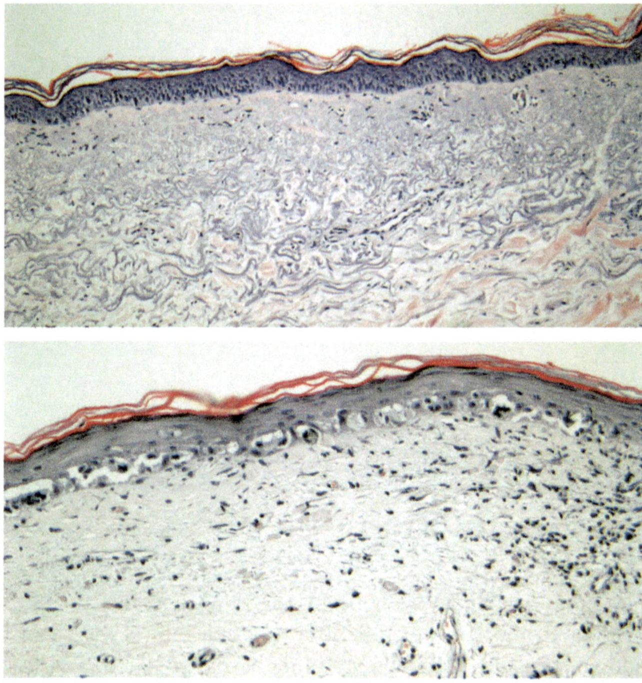

Fig. 1.1 *Bottom panel* reveals almost continuous single melanocyte proliferation in the epidermal basal layer, solar elastosis; diagnosis lentigo maligna. *Top panel* reveals less obvious basal melanocytic proliferation; diagnosis atypical JMH. In this case both panels are from the same patient's lesion of lentigo maligna. This illustrates the variability of the degree of melanocytic hyperplasia in one lesion and the importance of sampling a wide area of a lesion suspected as lentigo maligna

So What Is Atypical JMH?

Many times, the pathology report for a biopsy specimen in which the clinician suspected solar lentigo versus lentigo maligna carries the diagnosis of "atypical junctional melanocytic hyperplasia." This is a histological conceptual diagnosis and not a clinical diagnosis, at least not for the time being.

In order to understand this concept, it is important to go to the other end of the spectrum of junctional melanocytic proliferations, namely melanoma in situ.

The diagnosis of *melanoma in situ* is made with ease in biopsy specimens that reveal diffuse proliferation of uniformly atypical melanocytes (melanoma cells), at least in the basal layer with or without involvement of the outer epidermal layers. In most cases of the lentigo maligna type of melanoma in situ, the proliferation is limited to the basal layer; while in most cases of the superficial spreading type of melanoma in situ, the proliferation is throughout all layers of the epidermis.

The histological diagnosis of atypical JMH is generally made when the proliferation is more than simple JMH of a junctional or dysplastic nevus, but short of that in melanoma in situ.

So what is a practitioner to do?

The answer to this question requires a discussion of known causes with a report of atypical JMH.

Causes of Atypical JMH

The first is *severe chronic sun damage*. Biopsies of the skin of the face for other lesions in a patient with severe chronic sun damage often reveal junctional melanocyte proliferation, which is a common response of junctional melanocytes to chronic ultraviolet damage. This is commonly observed over fibrous papules, dermal nevi, and other face lesions, occasionally to such intensity as to overshadow the dermal pathology especially in incomplete superficial biopsy specimens. A pathologist may decide to report on it or not. Biopsy of normal-appearing adjacent skin would most likely reveal similar findings.

The second cause of atypical JMH is trauma, characteristically by a *recent surgical procedure*. Re-excision specimens of recently biopsied neoplasms often reveal junctional melanocytic proliferation that was not present in the original recent biopsy specimen and is believed to be secondary to the process of wound healing. This is often easy to identify over a new scar and is rarely reported on by the pathologist.

The third is *lentigo maligna*, which is sun-induced melanoma in situ with limited invasive potential. Lentigo maligna has displaced superficial spreading melanoma as the most common type of melanoma. Practitioners are well aware of the clinical appearance of a large, irregularly pigmented and irregularly bordered patch on chronically sun-exposed skin, especially the face. For the accurate histological diagnosis of lentigo maligna, an adequate-sized biopsy or multiple biopsies are often required. This is due to the fact that unlike other types of melanoma, the degree of proliferation is somewhat variable within the lesion. Where the proliferation is mild, the diagnosis may be missed and in the absence of characteristic findings of another identifiable melanocytic neoplasm, a pathologist may simply make the diagnosis of *atypical JMH*.

In the author's experience, a second or larger biopsy specimen of a lesion clinically suspected to be lentigo maligna often reveals characteristic findings that confirm the diagnosis. Hence, it is possible to avoid receiving the diagnosis of atypical JMH caused primarily by a small biopsy specimen of lentigo maligna if multiple small biopsies or preferably a wide biopsy is submitted initially.

Since patients with lentigo maligna are highly likely to have a background, or so-called field effect, of significant JMH due to severe sun damage, how is a surgeon or pathologist to determine *clear margins on a lentigo maligna excision* commonly performed by the staged Mohs technique?

This question is asked to pathologists on a regular basis. Lentigo maligna is characterized by almost continuous proliferation of single melanocytes in the basal layer compared to the ratio of one melanocyte for every six to eight basal cells in non-sun-exposed skin, and a larger ratio in sun-damaged skin. As successive layers of peripheral skin are removed by the Mohs technique, at what ratio should a pathologist be comfortable that the lentigo maligna has been completely excised?

There are no guidelines that help answer this question. Both, pathologists and dermatologic surgeons vary in their stringency of defining the borders of lentigo maligna, possibly explaining the occasional recurrence of lentigo maligna following Mohs surgical excision. Some pathologists use immunohistochemical markers to identify proliferating melanocytes.

It is reasonable to say that lentigo maligna should be excised to its border with background skin which, as mentioned above, highly likely has some degree of JMH due to chronic sun damage. But how is a pathologist to know the degree of this background melanocytic hyperplasia? In the author's experience, a 2–3 mm biopsy of normal-appearing skin of the contralateral side has been extremely helpful in identifying the degree of background melanocytic hyperplasia, especially in cases where the lentigo maligna "does not seem to end" after several layers of excision.

Conclusions

The term atypical JMH does not refer to a clinical lesion, but instead to a histological finding. A search for its cause is mandatory. This requires further biopsies or further evaluation by the pathologist and clinical correlation.

Chapter 2
What Is Dysplastic Nevus?

Figure 2.1 illustrates cases with disorders discussed in this chapter.

Definitions

What Is Dysplastic?

The dictionary defines dysplastic as an "abnormal growth or development of cells, tissue, bone, or organ."

What Is a Nevus?

The dictionary defines nevus as "any congenital anomaly of the skin, including moles and various types of birthmarks," or "any congenital growth or pigmented blemish on the skin; birthmark, or mole."

So What Is Dysplastic Nevus?

In 1978, the first report on what was named dysplastic nevus DN was published in the archives of dermatology by Wallace Clark and colleagues. The neoplasm was defined as a unique type of melanocytic nevus that occurred in two families with melanoma and multiple such nevi. Because the histological and clinical findings in the nevi of these patients were different from banal nevi, it was called DN, implying with unusual, atypical (or dysplastic) features. Soon after, similar lesions, clinically and histologically, were reported outside the familial melanoma setting, and called sporadic dysplastic nevi. Even in this nonfamilial setting, dysplastic nevi were found to increase a person's risk for melanoma independent of other melanoma risk factors.

D. F. Mutasim, *Practical Skin Pathology*, DOI 10.1007/978-3-319-14729-1_2

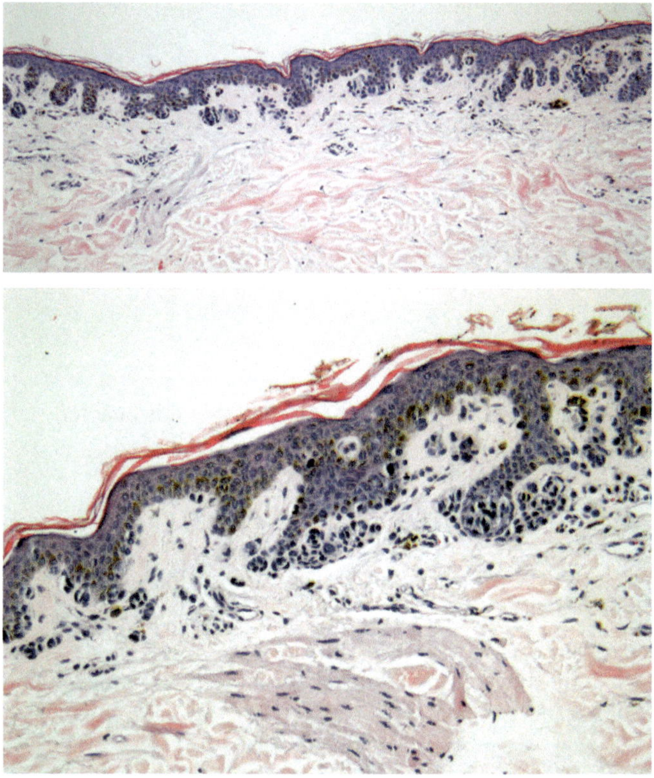

Fig. 2.1 *Top panel* reveals junctional proliferation of melanocytes in a predominantly nested pattern characteristic of junctional nevus. *Bottom panel* reveals that many melanocytes are hyperchromatic and that some nevus cells are seen along the shoulders of the rete, characteristic of the dysplastic nevus

Thus, the epidemic of the dysplastic nevus was born. Around 10% of the pathology material the author reads on a daily basis is to rule out dysplastic or atypical nevus. The neoplasm has progressively penetrated the awareness of the general public, in some cases producing fear in affected individuals, their friends, and relatives. Many times, a patient is told she had pre-melanoma or even early melanoma when the pathology report says "dysplastic nevus." So how is this nevus diagnosed? What are the defining characteristics of dysplastic nevus? Are they reliable? Are they valid? Are they clinical or histological?

What Are the Defining Characteristics of Dysplastic Nevus?

Clinically, DN has features of the ABCD of melanoma, well known to dermatologists, but are generally stable (hence with very little or no E). Histologically, the dysplasia or atypia is recognized both in the architecture of the proliferation as well as cytology of the nevus cells.

Architecturally, the proliferation is asymmetric and the junctional component of a compound dysplastic nevus extends beyond the dermal component laterally, resulting in the macular and papular components of a lesion. Additionally, junctional nevus nests occupy the sides or shoulders of the rete in addition to the tips which occurs in a banal nevus. Unlike in a banal nevus, nevus cells are also likely to be present as single units among the basal layer, so-called lentiginous melanocytic hyperplasia. A nevus cell may be present in the spinous layer but prominent pagetoid spread is not seen and should raise suspicion for melanoma. In a DN, the papillary dermis also reveals some changes. These include fibrosis, dilated capillaries, melanophages, and lymphocytes, altogether contributing to the pinkish appearance of many dysplastic nevi, especially those that are not pigmented.

In addition to the above architectural features of the dysplastic nevus, there may be cytological or nuclear atypia as well. Unlike in melanoma, the nuclear atypia is random, that is, not uniform among all the proliferating junctional nevus cells. In other words, the atypia is sporadic, affecting scattered individual nevus cells among otherwise unremarkable ones. The degree of atypia has been arbitrarily divided into mild, moderate, and severe.

Using the above criteria, the 1991 NIH consensus conference on dysplastic nevus declared that a non-banal junctional or compound nevus would be interpreted as:

1. With architectural disorder only.
2. With architectural disorder and cytological atypia. Then, the cytological atypia be graded as mild, moderate, or severe.

Most pathologists use either these criteria or personal modifications on them.

Are the Criteria Reliable? And Valid?

To the extent that the above features were used to define DN, they are valid, but not 100 % reliable. Interobserver agreement is far from 100 %, even among pathologists who practice together, and if read by the same pathologist at different times. Agreement improves, if the group of pathologists agrees in advance on strict diagnostic criteria to be used.

If criteria have been published, why is inter-observer agreement not 100%? Why does the diagnosis of such an important lesion seem subjective?

Architectural Disorder

How many of the above architectural disorder features should be present for a pathologist to diagnose architectural disorder? And how abnormal should each feature be in order to qualify?

Unfortunately, there are no answers to these questions, and it is left to the personal interpretation of each pathologist, contributing to the large degree of variability in diagnosis. Additionally, the so-called architectural disorder features are not unique to dysplastic nevi but some, such as melanophages, lymphocytes, and papillary dermal fibrosis, may be seen in early, otherwise unremarkable junctional nevus and lentigo simplex. Nevi in children and early-onset nevi in general often reveal features of architectural disorder. In my experience, general pathologists without training in skin pathology are more likely to exaggerate the degree of atypia.

Cytological Atypia

How many junctional nevus cells, or what percentage of the junctional nevus cells, should reveal nuclear atypia in order for a pathologist to call a nevus dysplastic? Is nuclear atypia in few nevus cells enough?

Unfortunately, there is no answer to this question. For the obvious reason of extreme biologic variability of neoplasms, it has been difficult to address this question.

How About Grading the Atypia?

As mentioned above, there are no reliably measurable criteria to determine whether atypia is mild, moderate, or severe. It is no different from determining whether epidermal hyperplasia, spongiosis, or a lymphocytic infiltrate is mild, moderate, or severe. Thus, it is common for two pathologists reading the same specimen (or the same pathologist evaluating the same specimen at two different times) to differ by at least one grade.

What if the Clinical Features of a Nevus Are Dysplastic but the Histological Findings Are Not?

This situation must happen often. At least one-half of the specimens submitted to rule out dysplastic nevus in the author's experience are banal junctional or compound nevi. Assuming that they looked clinically atypical, what is a clinician to do?

It has been observed that clinically atypical nevi without histological atypia are a risk factor for melanoma, just as nevi defined by the traditional histological criteria as dysplastic.

With this information in mind, why then continue to remove atypically appearing nevi and ask the pathologist to rule out or in dysplastic nevus? The answer to this question is in the mind of each dermatology practitioner and likely varies among practitioners.

What Should the Name Be? What's in a Name?

A few years following the first publication on dysplastic nevi in patients with familial melanoma debate as to the nature of these nevi ensued. Some, championed by Dr. A. B. Ackerman, expressed their disagreement with the term "dysplastic" based on the dictionary meaning of the word and its lack of specificity (see definition of the word "dysplastic" above).

It was stated by these authors that dysplastic nevus is extremely common, and may be the most common type of junctional or compound nevus. Many expressed the view that the dysplastic nevus is one step along the way of a progression of melanocytic proliferations, and that it often evolves into a common junctional or compound nevus. This view had strong support in the observation that the elderly rarely manifest dysplastic nevi.

So to honor Dr. Clark, Dr. Ackerman recommended that the neoplasm in question be referred to as Clark nevus akin to nevus of Reed and Spitz nevus. This term is used in some parts of the USA, especially the East Coast where Dr. Clark did his work. Others prefer the term "atypical nevus."

Whether dysplastic, atypical, or Clark's, there is a nevus with some clinical and histological characteristics that confers on its patient an increased risk for melanoma. These patients tend to be young, fair-skinned, and of northern European ancestry. The nevus tends to favor the trunk, especially the back and occasionally sun-protected skin of the buttocks, unlike banal nevi. Patients with these neoplasms, especially if multiple, are at higher risk for the development of melanoma and should be screened according to their degree of risk, which includes other well-known melanoma risk factors.

Should All Clinically Atypical-Appearing Nevi Be Biopsied?

There is a wide variation in practice among dermatologists.

On one hand, some (that may be called conservative) make the diagnosis of dysplastic nevus on clinical grounds, inform the patient that they are at increased risk for melanoma and recommend a screening schedule. They may obtain one or two biopsies at the initial visit to help support their clinical diagnosis. Many are skilled at using the dermatoscope, which helps them to suspect melanoma only in rare instances then performing biopsies.

On the other hand, some practitioners seem to remove every atypical appearing nevus. They probably base their practice on the fact that a dysplastic nevus is a potential precursor for melanoma, albeit very rarely.

How Should an Incompletely Excised DN Be Followed?

There are no universal recommendations to answer this question.

Studies based on questionnaires on the behavior of dermatologists in the USA show that the majority re-excise a nevus with cytologic atypia, especially if it is moderate or severe.

As accurate histological evaluation of a melanocytic neoplasm requires submitting the whole lesion, it may be a better clinical practice to ensure removal of the whole lesion at the time of biopsy.

Conclusions

For the foreseeable future, dermatologists will continue to face the questions about what to do when they see an atypical appearing nevus, and when they get a pathology report of dysplastic nevus (or other names implying the same).

Chapter 3
What Is Hypersensitivity Reaction?

Figure 3.1 illustrates a superficial and deep lymphocytic infiltrate.

Definition

Hypersensitivity is an immunological term that some pathologists have recently adopted as a histological diagnosis and some practitioners have started using clinically.

Immunologically speaking, hypersensitivity refers to the phenomenon in which certain predisposed individuals respond clinically to the antigens that the majority of individuals do not respond to. As such, immunological hypersensitivity is divided into four types.

Types of Hypersensitivity Reaction

Type I or anaphylaxis, is mediated by antigen, IgE antibody, and mast cells to produce hives and symptoms in other end organs, especially the respiratory tract. Acute allergic urticaria is the classic example.

Type II hypersensitivity reaction, also known as cytotoxic reaction, involves antigen–antibody interaction on the surface of cells such as red cells and platelets, resulting in anemia and thrombocytopenia. Autoimmune bullous disorders may be viewed as an example of type II reaction.

Type III hypersensitivity reaction, or immune complex disease spectrum, results from the deposition of antigen–antibody complexes on the endothelial cell surfaces of blood vessels or kidney, causing activation of complement, recruitment of inflammatory cells, and tissue destruction. Examples include many types of vasculitis and nephritis, including cutaneous leukocytoclastic vasculitis.

D. F. Mutasim, *Practical Skin Pathology*, DOI 10.1007/978-3-319-14729-1_3

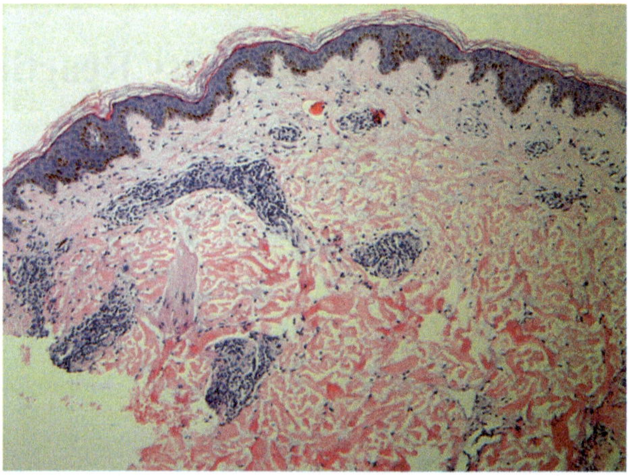

Fig. 3.1 The epidermis and papillary dermis are unremarkable. The reticular dermis reveals a perivascular lymphocytic infiltrate; thus, diagnosis as hypersensitivity reaction. In this case, an extensive search for a primary cause was nonrevealing; hence, the diagnosis of prurigo simplex was made

In serum sickness, animal-produced antibodies or antisera are injected into a patient with recent exposure to injurious antigen such as tetanus, resulting in antibody–antigen complexes that deposit in tissues, resulting in systemic inflammatory reaction. In the Arthus reaction, an animal gets repeatedly exposed locally to an antigen such as subcutaneous injections of horse serum, which result in an antibody response and a local immune reaction causing severe inflammation and sometimes gangrene at the site of injection.

Type IV hypersensitivity reaction, or cell-mediated immune response, refers to an antigen stimulating the cellular immune system namely T-lymphocytes, thus, resulting in activation and further recruitment of lymphocytes at the site of the reaction. A patient with a history of tuberculosis, unless extremely immune suppressed, has sensitized T-lymphocytes against the bacterial organism. The dermal injection of PPD containing the mycobacterial antigen recruits the specific lymphocytes that recruit further lymphocytes into the site of injection, resulting in an inflammatory response manifesting as redness and swelling. An individual with no previous exposure to tuberculosis would have no reaction.

So What Is Hypersensitivity Reaction for the Pathologist?

For those pathologists who use the term histologically including the author, there is no specific immunological correlation to the constellation of histological findings that they attribute to a "hypersensitivity reaction." In other words, the histological term does not refer to any specific immunological process. In general, the diagnosis of hypersensitivity reaction is given to an inflammatory reaction of the dermis, which does not conform to specific known inflammatory dermal disorders.

It is well known that the differential diagnosis of a primarily lymphocytic infiltrate of the reticular dermis is wide and includes tumid lupus erythematosus, benign lymphocytic infiltration of the skin, gyrate, or annular erythema (both superficial and deep), some drug eruptions, polymorphous light eruption, leukemia cutis, and so on.

If the infiltrate contains eosinophils, then the differential diagnosis is different and may include reaction to arthropod bite, scabies, urticaria, and pruritic urticarial papules and plaques of pregnancy (PUPPP). The histological findings in these four disorders have a high degree of overlap, and a specific diagnosis cannot be made in every case. When the lymphoeosinophilic infiltrate is not characteristic of any of the above disorders, a pathologist may feel compelled to give the descriptive interpretation of hypersensitivity reaction. The clinical lesion from which the biopsy is obtained is usually a red papule or plaque, and the practitioner often suspects the lesions to be the result of an allergic reaction to a local or systemic antigen; hence, it is appropriate to use the term hypersensitivity reaction histologically.

Whether the papules are caused by one of the above known papular disorders or are idiopathic (often referred to as prurigo simplex) is ultimately determined by the clinical practitioner based on further aspects of the history and physical examination.

Conclusions

A histological diagnosis of hypersensitivity reaction is not a final clinical diagnosis, rather an invitation to search for a possible cause.

Chapter 4
What Is Spongiotic Dermatitis?

Figure 4.1 illustrates severe spongiosis.

Dermatitis

The term *dermatitis* is used to denote different things for different people. For the dermatology *practitioner*, it refers to a group of clinical disorders that share features of papulovesicles in the acute phase, scaly patches in the subacute phase, and generally lichenified plaques in the chronic stage. It often is used for what others may call eczematous dermatitis. To the *general pathologist*, it often means an inflammatory noninfectious and nonneoplastic disorder of the skin.

For the *dermatopathologist*, dermatitis refers to a group of disorders in which pathology is limited to the epidermis and papillary dermis, and is further divided into three main categories (spongiotic, psoriasiform, and interface) based on the most prominent feature of the disorder (epidermal edema, epidermal hyperplasia, and disturbance of the dermo-epidermal junction, respectively).

Spongiotic Dermatitis

Spongiotic dermatitis refers to a group of disorders in which inflammation is focused on the epidermis and papillary dermis. Its hallmark is intercellular edema of the epidermis. This is associated with exocytosis of lymphocytes and a papillary dermal perivascular infiltrates of lymphocytes with or without eosinophils. In the *acute* phase, the spongiosis may be so severe that it can result in intraepidermal vesicles. In the *subacute* phase, the spongiosis decreases and the epidermis becomes hyperplastic, resulting in acanthosis and often parakeratosis. In the *chronic* phase, especially in the face of repeated scratching and or rubbing, epidermal hyperplasia progresses and the papillary dermis becomes thickened, resulting in lichenification.

D. F. Mutasim, *Practical Skin Pathology*, DOI 10.1007/978-3-319-14729-1_4

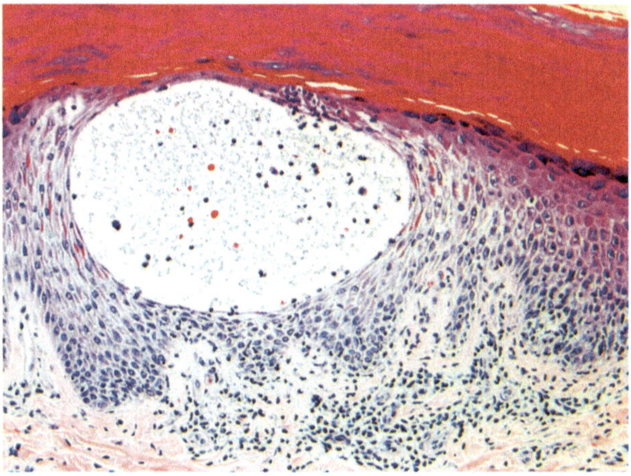

Fig. 4.1 Biopsy of acral skin lesion reveals marked spongiosis and intraepidermal vesicle in addition to a superficial lymphocytic infiltrate; thus, diagnosed as acute spongiotic dermatitis. In this case, the patient had "idiopathic" vesicular hand dermatitis, also known as dyshidrotic dermatitis and pompholyx

Spongiotic dermatitis may be allergic contact, atopic, nummular, stasis, photo-induced, and more. Certain histological clues may favor some forms of dermatitis over others. For example, the presence of so-called acute on chronic spongiotic dermatitis (referring to the combination of both epidermal hyperplasia and acute spongiosis) is characteristic of nummular dermatitis and chronic allergic contact dermatitis. Lichenification is more likely to be seen in patients with atopic dermatitis. The presence of prominent stasis changes in the papillary dermis underlying spongiotic epidermis raises strong suspicion for stasis dermatitis.

In general, a practitioner would not expect the pathologist to "type" the dermatitis but instead confirm the diagnosis to the exclusion of other disorders. On the other hand, an overzealous pathologist may attempt to make a specific diagnosis when the findings are simply those of spongiotic dermatitis. It is the practitioner's duty to diagnose the type of dermatitis of the patient based on the history and physical examination.

Special Types of Spongiotic Dermatitis

These are disorders that do not appear as dermatitis to the practitioner, yet reveale spongiosis on histological evaluation; so, this should be excluded before the histological diagnosis of spongiotic dermatitis is taken as evidence that the patient has clinical dermatitis. Fortunately, there are clues that often help the clinician and the pathologist to suspect these disorders.

Dermatitic or Eczematous Drug Eruption

Eczematous drug eruption presents as an acute, generalized red eruption a few days to weeks following the intake of the offending drug. It is generally easy to suspect as a drug reaction. Although many have suggested the presence of eosinophils as a helpful clue to a drug reaction eosinophils are also present in allergic contact, nummular, and atopic dermatitis. The pathophysiology of eczematous drug eruption is akin to that of allergic contact dermatitis, except that the exposure to the antigen is systemic rather than topical.

Pityriasis rosea

Pityriasis rosea (*PR*) is interesting in belonging to the "papulosquamous" group of disorders clinically (along with psoriasis, LP, and secondary syphilis), yet belongs to the spongiotic group histologically. The acute onset, mostly asymptomatic nature and pattern of the eruption, make the clinical diagnosis easy.

Histological clues to its diagnosis include mounded foci of parakeratosis, rare dyskeratosis, mild red cell extravasation, and generally mild spongiosis. Only rarely is the spongiosis moderate or severe. It is often possible to miss making the diagnosis histologically, so including PR in the clinical differential diagnosis is important.

Nutritional Disorders

Nutritional disorders vary more greatly in their clinical findings than histological findings. In general, epidermal dysmaturation and pallor raise a flag in the mind of the pathologist, especially in the absence of another specific diagnosis. When informed of the clinician's suspicion, a pathologist is most likely to be helpful.

Photodermatitis

Photodermatitis may be divided histologically into spongiotic and lichenoid; and etiologically into contact and systemic. When a contact or systemic agent causes photodermatitis, it is like a contactant or systemic medication causing spongiotic dermatitis (allergic contact and dermatitic drug eruption, respectively), except that ultraviolet light is needed as well.

Photodermatitis due to a systemic agent has been divided into phototoxic and photoallergic types, just as contact dermatitis is either irritant or allergic. The distinction, however, is not always possible and there is great overlap between the drugs that cause phototoxic and photoallergic eruptions. Hence, except in a few instances of clear phototoxicity (such as to the "cyclines"), drug-induced photo-eruption is best called photodermatitis or photosensitive dermatitis.

As such, the histology of photodermatitis is that of acute or subacute spongiotic dermatitis with occasional possible clues. These include dyskeratosis (in this setting also called sunburn cells), and a tendency for the lymphocytic infiltrate to extend beyond the papillary dermis into the superficial reticular dermis.

The discussion of photodermatitis would not be complete without addressing *chronic actinic dermatitis* (*CAD*). This term applies to a different form of photosensitivity characterized by a subacute to chronic dermatitis that is photodistributed and persistent. Patients are extremely sensitive to UVA light. The term CAD has been accepted as an umbrella diagnosis for three disorders with common features; namely, persistent light reaction, actinic reticuloid, and photosensitive eczema. Unlike patients with drug-induced photodermatitis in whom discontinuation of the offending drug usually results in resolution of the eruption, patients with CAD generally have a worse morbidity and are more difficult to treat.

The histopathology of chronic actinic dermatitis is that of subacute to chronic (photo)dermatitis, rarely mimicking mycosis fungoides, especially in the actinic reticuloid subtype.

Fungal and Yeast Infections

A histological clue that spongiotic dermatitis may be caused by a fungal or yeast infection is the presence of neutrophils in the horny layer. Special stains often confirm the diagnosis unless a fungal infection has been partially treated.

Paraneoplastic

One of the clinical causes of the histological diagnosis of spongiotic dermatitis is erythroderma or exfoliative dermatitis; and one of the causes of exfoliative dermatitis is underlying malignancy, especially of the lymphoproliferative type, chief among them may be Hodgkin's lymphoma. In the setting of erythroderma in which the histopathology is that of spongiotic dermatitis to the exclusion of psoriasis, pityriasis rubra pilaris (PRP), and Sezary syndrome, underlying lymphoma should be considered.

Mycosis Fungoides

MF is a great mimicker clinically and histologically. One of the histological patterns of patch and plaque MF is spongiotic. Occasionally, the spongiosis is so severe that it may overshadow the epidermotropism, and the diagnosis may be missed.

I have seen several patients who carried the diagnosis of eczematous dermatitis for years before the diagnosis of MF was made. These are generally older individuals with "resistant dermatitis." Clinical suspicion of MF and obtaining a biopsy is highly valuable in this setting.

Conclusions

Most biopsies interpreted histologically as "spongiotic dermatitis" reflect disorders that are clinically "dermatitis." There are, however, other disorders that reveal the histology of spongiotic dermatitis, yet do not belong to the group of "dermatitides" but instead to infections, papulosquamous disorders, neoplasms, and paraneoplastic disorders. Close cooperation between the clinician and the pathologist is essential in making the right diagnosis.

Chapter 5
What Is Psoriasiform Dermatitis?

Figure 5.1 demonstrates orthohyperkeratosis, acanthosis, and papillary dermal fibrosis.

What Is Psoriasiform Dermatitis?

Psoriasiform dermatitis is a histological term that refers to a group of disorders that histologically mimic psoriasis. Chief among them in frequency are lichenified dermatitis or lichen simplex chronicus (LSC), seborrheic dermatitis, and pityriasis rubra pilaris (PRP). Secondary syphilis and mycosis fungoides (MF) may both reveal findings of psoriasiform dermatitis among their many histological presentations.

So What Are Those Findings?

For a biopsy specimen to be interpreted as psoriasiform dermatitis it must have the following findings, which are usually characteristic of plaque psoriasis, albeit to a lesser degree (otherwise they would represent psoriasis):

- Epidermal hyperplasia that tends toward regular and favors the rete
- Parakeratosis
- No or at the best, mild spongiosis

Other findings may include neutrophils in the horny layer, exocytosis, and a superficial infiltrate.

It is primarily the regular epidermal hyperplasia that pathologists require for labeling a dermatitis psoriasiform. Some use the term psoriasiform as an adjective for the epidermal hyperplasia rather than for the dermatitis, speaking of psoriasiform epidermal hyperplasia to mean regular epidermal hyperplasia like in plaque psoriasis.

D. F. Mutasim, *Practical Skin Pathology*, DOI 10.1007/978-3-319-14729-1_5

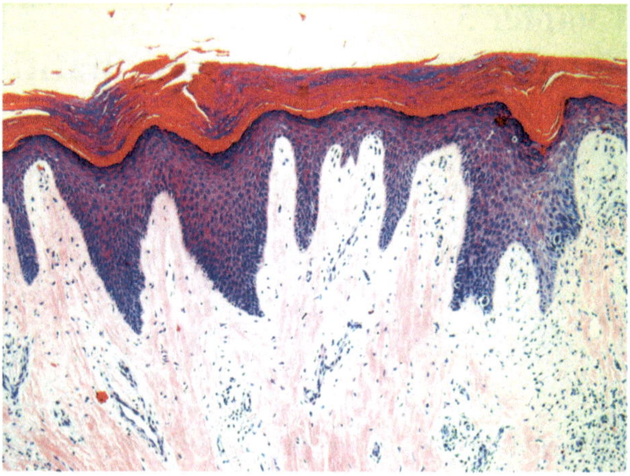

Fig. 5.1 Biopsy from a solitary plaque of LSC reveals compact ortho-hyperkeratosis, marked epidermal hyperplasia, and fibrosis of the superficial dermis along with a mild lymphocytic infiltrate

Clinical Disorders with Histological Findings of Psoriasiform Dermatitis

Disorders in this group include

- LSC
- PRP
- seborrheic dermatitis
- secondary syphilis
- MF, and
- inflammatory linear verrucous epidermal nevus ILVEN

These disorders do not share clinical findings or common etiology.

Histological Clues

Compared to the characteristic findings of stable plaque *psoriasis* (namely, diffuse parakeratosis with collections of neutrophils, loss of the granular layer, moderate to severe regular elongation of the rete with atrophy of the suprapapillary component of the epidermis, exocytosis of neutrophils, tortuous capillaries in the dermal papillae, and a superficial lymphocytic infiltrate), lesions of chronic lichenified atopic dermatitis and *LSC* tend to have more orthohyperkeratosis, intact or thick granular layer, hyperplasia of both the rete and inter-rete epidermis, and thickening of the papillary dermis, along with a superficial infiltrate.

PRP has some features of lichenified dermatitis and others of psoriasis. Instead of diffuse parakeratosis, there is alternating orthokeratosis and parakeratosis in both the horizontal and the vertical plane of the horny layer, mild to moderate epidermal hyperplasia that is not as regular as in psoriasis. Primary follicular papules are more common in PRP than in psoriasis.

Seborrheic dermatitis is probably the most difficult disorder in this section to differentiate from psoriasis. So much so that pathologists and clinicians alike have recognized and named a disorder that appears clinically and histologically intermediate between seborrheic dermatitis and psoriasis, namely *sebopsoriasis*. Different authors have used the term for different findings; some for (usually exuberant) seborrheic dermatitis in a patient with psoriasis, others for psoriasis in the seborrheic region.

Secondary syphilis is often easily suspected when the infiltrate contains abundant plasma cells and or histiocytes and if, in addition to the psoriasiform pattern of epidermal hyperplasia, there are interface changes as well. Extension of the infiltrate into the deep dermis is a strong clue to the diagnosis of syphilis.

MF commonly has a psoriasiform appearance at scanning magnification. The presence of single or grouped lymphocytes with clear halos around them especially in the basal layer easily points to the diagnosis.

Finally, *ILVEN* may be so psoriasiform histologically that it has been considered by some in the past as a form of linear psoriasis. Evidence since then has indicated that ILVEN is a unique disorder. Small foci of parakeratosis alternate with orthokeratosis on a regular basis. The granular layer is lost beneath the foci of parakeratosis, and the epidermis is moderately to severely hyperplastic in a regular pattern. The combination of these findings in the proper clinical setting is diagnostic of ILVEN.

Conclusions

What May a Practitioner Do with a Pathology Report That Simply Says Psoriasiform Dermatitis? It is fair to expect that a diagnosis of psoriasiform dermatitis is accompanied by a differential diagnosis and the degree of likelihood of each of the suspected disorders. If the report does not include such a differential diagnosis, the practitioner may call the pathologist and ask for one. If a clinical differential diagnosis has been submitted on the requisition form, the pathologist is more likely to address the likelihood of each of the disorders; hence, the importance of providing clinical information to the pathologist.

Chapter 6
What Is Lichenoid Dermatitis?

Figure 6.1 demonstrates hyperkeratosis, focal hypergranulosis, and a diffuse lymphocytic infiltrate.

What Is Lichenoid Dermatitis?

In classifying the various inflammatory disorders of the skin by their patterns, interface dermatitis refers to the disorders in which the primary site of pathology is the interface between the epidermis and the dermis; that is, the dermo–epidermal junction. Interface dermatitis is then divided into two subgroups: vacuolar and lichenoid.

The prototype of vacuolar interface dermatitis is erythema multiforme, and the features are:

- Basal vacuolization (also known as hydropic degeneration or vacuolar degeneration of basal cells)
- Variable dyskeratosis
- Superficial lymphocytic infiltrate

The prototype of lichenoid interface dermatitis is lichen planus (LP) and the histological features are:

- A band-like, usually dense lymphocytic infiltrate in the papillary dermis that obscures the dermo–epidermal junction
- Squamatization of basal cells, that is, basal cells lose their identifiable features and instead become larger with evidence of squamous differentiation (more deeply eosinophilic cytoplasm like differentiated keratinocytes), a phenomenon that has been referred to also as premature keratinization/cornification, and manifests histologically as dyskeratosis
- Epidermal hyperplasia with characteristic saw-tooth appearance to the rete, hypergranulosis, and compact orthokeratosis

D. F. Mutasim, *Practical Skin Pathology*, DOI 10.1007/978-3-319-14729-1_6

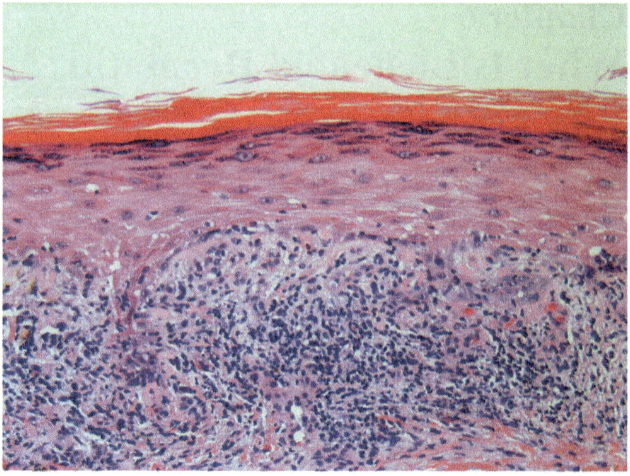

Fig. 6.1 Moderately compact orthohyperkeratosis, hypergranulosis, mild acanthosis, saw-toothing of the tips of the rete, few dyskeratotic basal cells, and a band-like lymphocytic infiltrate are characteristic of lichen planus

Lichenoid dermatitis or lichenoid interface dermatitis, is a histological term used for referring to a combination of histological findings close to those of LP. Disorders in this category include those with a superficial infiltrate and disorders in which the infiltrate may extend to the deep plexus. The former include

- lichenoid drug eruption (which is often photoinduced)
- lichen nitidus
- lichenoid keratosis
- lichenoid capillaritis (lichen aureus)
- lichenoid mycosis fungoides MF
- pityriasis lichenoides chronica PLC, and
- keratosis lichenoides chronica KLC.

The latter include lichenoid lupus erythematosus and lichen striatus.

So Is Lichenoid Dermatitis a Legitimate Diagnosis to Provide on a Pathology Report?

Not if there is no histological differential diagnosis and degree of likelihood of each diagnosis. Most of the above disorders have characteristic histological findings that, with some clinical information, a diagnosis should be made in most cases. The findings in lichen nitidus, lichenoid keratosis, lichen aureus, lichenoid MF, and lichen striatus are so characteristic that reporting their findings here is unnecessary.

The disorders that the author has seen not diagnosed histologically with certainty are lichenoid photodermatitis, PLC, KLC, and lichenoid subacute lupus erythematosus. Patients who have been referred with one of these disorders often brought pathology reports that simply were interpreted as "lichenoid dermatitis."

Addressing the Difficulties

What is the relationship between drug-induced lichen planus, lichen planus-like drug eruption, lichenoid drug eruption, and lichenoid photodermatitis? Are these distinct disorders or are they related? There is no perfect agreement in the literature as to the answer.

In the author's view, drug-induced lichen planus and lichen planus-like drug eruption are forms of lichen planus that are induced by some drug (classic among the list is gold). The clinical presentation is indistinguishable from otherwise idiopathic lichen planus, just as the clinical picture of drug-induced superficial pemphigus is indistinguishable from that of idiopathic superficial pemphigus, and the clinical picture of drug-induced urticaria is indistinguishable from idiopathic urticaria or urticaria secondary to other agents.

So Are There Histological Features that May Raise Suspicion for Drug Etiology in a Patient with Lichen Planus?

It had been reported that the presence of foci of parakeratosis and eosinophils among the lymphocytic infiltrate strongly suggest drug etiology. This is true when comparing groups of patients but cannot be applied to individual cases. Some patients with LP and eosinophils and/or parakeratosis have not been taking any medication.

How About Lichenoid Drug Eruption and Lichenoid Photodermatitis?

Strictly speaking, the first term applies to an eruption that is drug-induced with histological findings of lichenoid interface dermatitis. If the findings are those of lichen planus, this term should then be replaced with drug-induced lichen planus. If the lichenoid features histologically, however are subtle, then the term lichenoid drug eruption is appropriate. In the author's experience, the eruptions in most patients in whom a drug has caused a lichenoid eruption has been photodistributed; hence, the term lichenoid photodermatitis may be more appropriate. In the author's experience as well as in the literature, most of these patients are dark skinned and are highly sensitive to UVA light as detected by phototesting.

What About Lichenoid Lupus Erythematosus?

Lupus erythematosus (LE) is among the group of vacuolar interface dermatitis (prototype erythema multiforme). There is prominent vacuolar degeneration of basal cells without their obliteration by a band-like interface lymphocytic infiltrate, in addition to the superficial and deep perivascular and periadnexal infiltrate. Some cases, however, may have an interface lymphocytic infiltrate as well. Such cases have been referred to as lichenoid LE. These patients have clinical lesions of either discoid LE or subacute LE. A clinical feature that may raise suspicion for lichenoid DLE is the tendency for the red color of DLE to have a violaceous hue.

What Is Lupus/Lichen Planus Overlap?

The term overlap is used in dermatology when an eruption has features of more than one disorder. In some cases, a new term is given for an eruption with overlap features. For example, the overlap of lichen planus and pemphigoid has been named lichen planus pemphigoides. Lesions of each disorder coexist in the same patient and overlap in the same area of skin. Similarly, morphea and lichen sclerosis may coexist both as separate lesions in the same patient or may coexist in the same lesion.

For the diagnosis of lupus lichen planus overlap to be made, a patient must have clinical, histological, and immunofluorescence findings of both disorders separately and/or together. A high clinical index of suspicion is required, and multiple biopsies may be needed.

The distinction between lichenoid LE and LP/LE overlap is not always clear in the literature.

How About Mycosis Fungoides? Capillaritis? Secondary Syphilis?

Each of these three disorders has multiple histological presentations, one of which is lichenoid. There are clues to making each diagnosis. In secondary syphilis, in addition to the superficial infiltrate there is often a deeper infiltrate, and in addition to lymphocytes, plasma cells, and/or histiocytes are often present. In lichenoid capillaritis or lichen aureus, the infiltrate tends to be strikingly band-like and dense, filling the papillary dermis. Red cells and/or siderophages help confirm the diagnosis. Lichenoid MF may be missed histologically if epidermotropism is overshadowed by the dense and diffuse infiltrate, but is suspected if characteristic findings of other lichenoid disorders are missing.

How About PLC and KLC?

The textbook findings of PLC are seen in mature red finely scaly flat-topped thin papules. An early or late lesion of PLC may have uncharacteristic histological findings, and the diagnosis may be missed. In such cases, the pathology report may simply indicate lichenoid dermatitis. Hence, the importance of obtaining multiple biopsies in patients suspected to have PLC.

KLC is rarely suspected by pathologists due to its rarity and lack of unique characteristics. Lesions of KLC have "incomplete" lichenoid interface features, that is, an interface infiltrate that is not band-like, and epidermal hyperplasia that is somewhat akin to psoriasiform epidermal hyperplasia. A histological diagnosis of KLC requires an extremely high index of suspicion and/or alerting the pathologist that the disorder is being considered clinically.

Conclusions

The histological diagnosis of lichenoid dermatitis is a beginning rather than an end. A search for the underlying clinical disorder requires efforts by both the clinical practitioner and the pathologist.

Chapter 7
What Is Granulomatous Dermatitis?

Figure 7.1 illustrates a focus of dermal degeneration surrounded by a histiocte-rich infiltrate.

Definition

Unlike the term "dermatitis" as used by dermatology practitioners and dermatopathologists to refer to superficial skin pathology involving the epidermis and papillary dermis and that may be spongiotic, interface, or psoriasiform; the use of the term dermatitis in "granulomatous dermatitis" is loose. It simply refers to a process in the skin in which the infiltrate is granulomatous, that is, primarily histiocytic the term is used by general pathologists more than dermatopathologists.

Histiocyte

A histiocyte is a differentiated tissue monocyte. Histiocyte is the agreed-upon name for a cell that had carried few other names as being part of the immune system (monocyte–phagocyte system, reticulo–endothelial system, and lymphoreticular system).

A histiocyte may be a macrophage (expressing its ability to phagocytose organisms and foreign matter) or dendritic cell (a cell that processes and presents antigen). The epidermal Langerhans cell is another differentiated monocyte.

Histiocyte in Skin Pathology

A few undifferentiated monocytes may be present in a primarily lymphocytic infiltrate. These are hard to differentiate from lymphocytes under light microscopy. When a monocyte becomes a histiocyte it acquires phagocytic function and mor-

D. F. Mutasim, *Practical Skin Pathology*, DOI 10.1007/978-3-319-14729-1_7

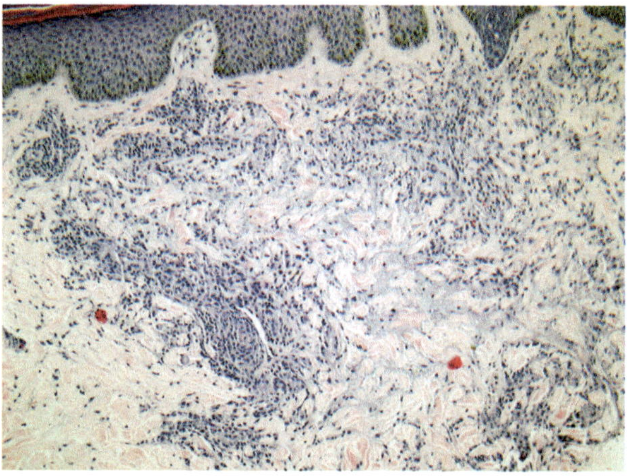

Fig. 7.1 Beneath an unremarkable epidermis, a focus of basophilic degeneration of collagen is surrounded in a palisading manner by histiocytes and lymphocytes characteristic of granuloma annulare

phological characteristics that makes it easily detectable by routine histology. It becomes larger, its cytoplasm abundant, and often acquires an Idaho potato appearance, or it becomes an "epithelioid cell," meaning, it becomes rounded and closely packed with other similar cells resembling epithelial cells. Organisms such as leprosy organisms or material such as lipid, melanin, or iron may be visible in its cytoplasm, so it may be called a lepra cell, xanthoma cell, melanophage, or siderophage.

Histiocytes in Granulomatous Inflammation

An infiltrate is granulomatous if it is abundant in histiocytes, especially if the histiocytes form collections, so-called granulomas.

Granulomas are further divided etiologically into infectious, inflammatory, and foreign body granulomas; and divided histologically into sarcoidal, tuberculoid, palisading, and suppurative granulomas, with great overlap among and between the two groups.

Sarcoidal Granuloma

A granuloma is named sarcoidal if it is similar to the granuloma of sarcoidosis; namely, a collection of epithelioid histiocytes generally containing very few adjacent lymphocytes, and a variable number of multinucleated cells. Central granuloma necrosis is rare or nonexistent.

The differential diagnosis of sarcoidal granuloma is *sarcoidosis*, *granulomatous rosacea* (granulomatous rosacea may also be tuberculoid or mixed), *granulomatous cheilitis, ectopic Crohn disease,* some kinds of *foreign body reaction such as to silica or tattoo,* and multiple dermal cutaneous *infections,* including tuberculoid leprosy, and established lesions of atypical mycobacterial infections, *Leishmania*, and many fungi.

When an infectious organism or a foreign body is not detected in a sarcoidal granuloma, clinical pathological correlation is necessary and usually straightforward except in biopsies from the face, where the differential diagnosis includes papular sarcoidosis and granulomatous rosacea. These require further clinical examination for facial and extrafacial evidence of both diseases.

Tuberculoid Granuloma

In contrast to sarcoidal granuloma, a tuberculoid granuloma is generally rich in lymphocytes, often reveals central caseation necrosis, and may contain Langhans giant cells. The differential diagnosis of tuberculoid granuloma includes some forms of *cutaneous tuberculosis, rosacea, and many infections.*

Palisading Granuloma

In disorders characterized by palisading granuloma, there is a central zone of degenerated collagen surrounded by histiocytes and other inflammatory cells in a radiating or palisading manner. The three prototypic examples are *granuloma annulare (GA), necrobiosis lipoidica (NL), and rheumatoid nodule.* They differ by the size, degree, and staining characteristics of the degenerated collagen in the center; and, by the type and pattern of the surrounding infiltrate, and are easy to differentiate.

Suppurative Granuloma

Suppurative granuloma occurs in disorders in which there are both an acute suppurative neutrophilic abscess and an adjacent chronic histiocytic/granulomatous process. Suppurative granuloma is characteristic of foreign body reaction such as to splinter or to ruptured hair follicle (such as in *acne, folliculitis decalvans, and dissecting cellulitis*), and multiple chronic *infections*, including fungal infections like sporotrichosis and blastomycosis, atypical mycobacterial infections, such as *Mycobacterium marinum* and *Leishmania.*

Some authors propose a fifth type of granuloma that they name foreign body granuloma. Depending on the type of foreign body and the age of the lesion, a foreign body granuloma may appear suppurative, suppurative granulomatous, or sarcoidal; hence, was not considered here separately.

Conclusions

The differential diagnosis of granulomatous dermal inflammation is wide and is classified both by etiology and pattern of infiltrate. In cases that cannot be confirmed based on the histological evaluation alone, special stains for organisms and polarization for some foreign bodies as well as cultures are indicated.

Chapter 8
What Is Dermatitis with Epidermotropism?

Figure 8.1 illustrates several single hyperchromatic lymphocytes in the epidermis, without spongiosis.

What Is Epidermotropism?

As the name implies, epidermotropism refers to the phenomenon of lymphocytes residing in the epidermis. This is in contrast to exocytosis, in which lymphocytes move out through the epidermis. Exocytosis is associated with spongiosis while epidermotropism is associated with clear halos around individual lymphocytes and generally lacks spongiosis. While exocytosis and spongiosis are characteristic features of inflammatory disorders, such as eczematous dermatitis, epidermotropism is characteristic of mycosis fungoides (MF), the most common type of cutaneous T-cell lymphoma (CTCL).

What, Besides Mycosis Fungoides, May Have Epidermotropism?

The disorders are

- lymphomatoid drug eruption
- lymphomatoid papulosis and
- non-MF CTCL, such as aggressive cytotoxic CD8+ epidermotropic TCL, and
- adult T-leukemia lymphoma ATLL.

All these disorders may have significant epidermotropism and be misdiagnosed as mycosis fungoides.

D. F. Mutasim, *Practical Skin Pathology*, DOI 10.1007/978-3-319-14729-1_8

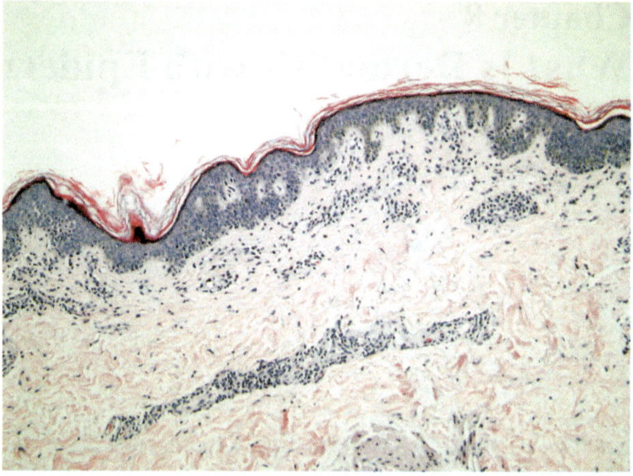

Fig. 8.1 A nonspecific mild superficial perivascular lymphocytic infiltrate accompanies epidermis with several discrete lymphocytes with clear halos within the basal layer, characteristic of mycosis fungoides

Is Epidermotropism Always Easy to Identify?

The answer is no. In early lesions of mycosis fungoides, the intraepidermal lymphocytes may be so few that they may be overlooked. Sometimes spongiosis accompanies epidermotropism and may overshadow it, resulting in making the wrong diagnosis of spongiotic dermatitis. This is especially true when the clinical presentation of mycosis fungoides is eczematous, and the clinician has not suspected the diagnosis in order to put it on the requisition form. The author has seen several such cases managed for a long time as eczematous dermatitis.

Histological Clues

Most lesions of *patch and plaque MF* have characteristic histological findings and are easily diagnosed. Difficulties arise under the following conditions:

1. If there is significant concomitant spongiosis
2. In very early lesions previously called *pre-mycotic* disorders; that is, disorders with the capacity to transform into mycosis fungoides. *Parapsoriasis* (discussed elsewhere) was paramount among them. Other disorders were chronic persistent dermatitis or chronic superficial dermatitis.

Whether parapsoriasis and related disorders are potential precursors for MF just as an actinic keratosis is a potential precursor for squamous cell carcinoma or whether they are the earliest manifestation of MF, has been debated for a few decades in both the USA and Europe. There is almost a general agreement now that they are early forms of mycosis fungoides, and their names may be discontinued.

Some clinicians may find it useful to retain the term parapsoriasis to avoid using a malignant term such as MF or CTCL for a patient who has one or two stable patches of long duration, and in whom survival is known to be similar to individuals with no such lesions. Use of the term parapsoriasis not only alleviates the anxiety associated with a diagnosis of malignant disorder, but also avoids the patient having difficulty obtaining life insurance.

One should keep in mind that the initial use of the word parapsoriasis around 100 years ago was to apply to a group of disorders that did not belong to the (then recognized) inflammatory conditions of the skin, and which shared with psoriasis its chronic nature, lack of symptoms, and general lack of response to (then available) treatments.

Lymphomatoid drug eruption, also known as MF-like drug eruption, is a type of drug eruption whose histological findings mimic those of mycosis fungoides, namely having some degree of epidermotropism. In addition to epidermotropism, there is a strong tendency for mild spongiosis, so if the diagnosis of lymphomatoid drug eruption is missed histologically, the findings would either have been interpreted as mycosis fungoides or spongiotic dermatitis. Moreover, the clinical presentation of lymphomatoid drug eruption is also variable and may present as subacute dermatitis-like patches to reddish papules and plaques to exfoliative erythroderma.

The diagnosis should be considered histologically if the pathologist suspects MF but feels that the combination of findings is not strong enough to confirm the diagnosis. Discontinuation of the offending drug, followed by resolution of eruption in a few weeks to a few months should confirm the diagnosis.

Lymphomatoid papulosis (*LyP*) is both clinically and histologically heterogenous. Although the original description of the disorder emphasized ulcerating nodules which healed with scars, the term was also later applied to papular lesions, which in some cases occurred in patients with MF. The so-called histological type A LyP, characteristic of the nodular lesions, reveals a moderately dense superficial and deep-mixed infiltrate of lymphocytes, histiocytes, eosinophils, and scattered large lymphocytes that label with antibodies to CD30, a lymphocyte activation marker. Type A LyP may be confused with insect bite reaction.

On the other hand, so-called type B LyP shares the histology of patch and plaque MF. Lesions of this type often occur in patients with MF, but follow the expected course of LyP, that is, spontaneous resolution. Without clinical history, it is not possible to differentiate histologically between the two disorders.

Non-MF cutaneous T-cell lymphomas, particularly aggressive cytotoxic CD8+epidermotropic TCL and ATLL, may be differentiated from MF by clinical findings and histologically by immunophenotyping. For practical purposes, if a biopsy specimen is reported as MF to the surprise of the practitioner due to lack of good clinicopathological correlation, then further evaluation of the histological findings is mandatory in order to consider the possibility of the other two disorders.

Conclusions

Although epidermotropism is characteristic of MF, it may be seen in several other disorders with different biological behavior and prognosis, so an accurate diagnosis is essential.

Chapter 9
What Is Drug Eruption?

Figure 9.1 illustrates a sparse lymphocytic infiltrate in the papillary dermis.

Definition

Simply put, a drug eruption is a skin eruption caused by a medication or drug. So is it appropriate to use the term "drug eruption" alone clinically and/or histologically? A strong case can be made that the answer should be "no."

Introduction

An eruption due to a medication may mimic most primary skin eruptions, e.g., urticaria, erythema multiforme (EM), pityriasis rosea (PR), psoriasis, panniculitis, bullous disorder, lichen planus (LP), dermatitis, and more. Hence, the term drug eruption should always be associated with the morphological type of the eruption. For example, urticarial drug eruption, pityriasis rosea-like drug eruption, drug-induced erythema multiforme, and eczematous drug eruption, among many others.

The histopathology of each of these drug eruptions is generally similar to that of the primary eruption, whether due to herpes virus infection for erythema multiforme, food allergy for urticaria, or systemic fungal infection for panniculitis.

Histological Clues

Some histological features may raise suspicion that an eruption may be due to a medication rather than idiopathic or due to other causes. None of these features, however, are diagnostic of drug etiology.

D. F. Mutasim, *Practical Skin Pathology*, DOI 10.1007/978-3-319-14729-1_9

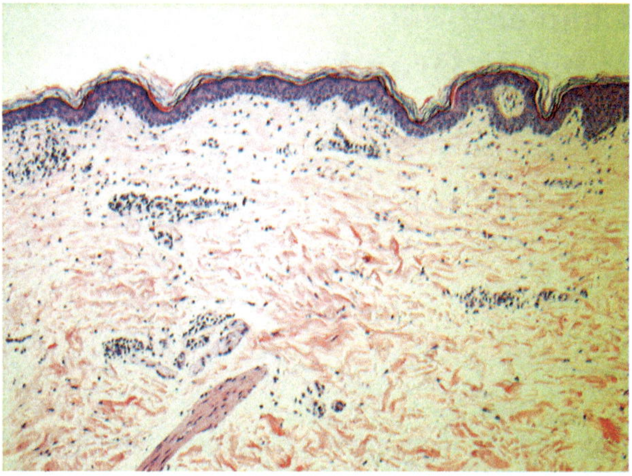

Fig. 9.1 A mild superficial perivascular lymphocytic infiltrate that focally approaches the dermo–epidermal junction is characteristic of morbilliform drug eruption as well as exanthem. In this case, the patient had a generalized macular eruption secondary to medication

The histological characteristics of *LP*, for example, are well known (compact orthohyperkeratosis, hypergranulosis, saw-tooth appearance of the rete, and a usually dense band-like lymphocytic infiltrate in the papillary dermis that obscures the epidermal basal layer and dermal epidermal junction). Drug-induced lichen planus (or lichen planus-like drug eruption) may have identical features to idiopathic lichen planus but may have foci of parakeratosis and some eosinophils among the lymphocytes. This conclusion was drawn from comparing biopsy specimens from a group of patients with idiopathic lichen planus to a group with drug-induced lichen planus. The correlation between the medication etiology and the two histological features was not absolute. Instead, there was an overlap in the histological findings between idiopathic and drug-induced LP.

In practice, a pathologist is likely to raise the possibility of a drug etiology for a case of LP, which demonstrates parakeratosis and/or eosinophils, and is unlikely to bring up the possibility of drug etiology in the absence of both findings; hence, circumventing a search for drug etiology. I believe it is the responsibility of the clinician more than the pathologist to suspect and determine if a case of LP is idiopathic or drug-induced.

In the case of *EM*, severe dyskeratosis and lesser infiltrate are more likely to be associated with drug rather than herpes virus etiology.

Whether *urticaria* is idiopathic, autoimmune, caused by a food allergy, or a medication cannot be determined by histological examination. A perivascular and interstitial infiltrate of lymphocytes and eosinophils is seen in all above types of urticaria. Sometimes the term *urticarial drug eruption* is used instead of drug-induced urticaria to refer to an eruption caused by a medication in which the lesions are edematous; hence, urticarial but not transient, like urticaria. In such cases, the infiltrate tends to be more superficial and may extend to the overlying epidermis, reminiscent of *urticarial dermatitis*.

Drug-induced dermatitis (*eczematous drug eruption*), *drug-induced pemphigus*, *drug-induced or aggravated psoriasis*, and *pityriasis rosea-like drug eruption* all cannot be differentiated histologically from the idiopathic disorder that they mimic.

How about generalized *morbilliform drug eruption*? The clinical differential diagnosis of morbilliform drug eruption is generally a viral exanthema, and less frequently mild, acute graft versus host disease. The pathologist is often faced with the question to differentiate between the two or three disorders, especially in hospitalized patients. The presence of eosinophils is used by many pathologists to support the diagnosis of drug eruption. The frequency with which eosinophils occur in morbilliform drug eruption, however, is not known and to what extent eosinophils may be present in viral exanthem is also not known. Hence, the use of eosinophils as a marker for drug eruption may not be accurate.

Many times, a dermatologist submits a biopsy requisition form with "rule out drug eruption" and sometimes a pathology report may have as a diagnosis "drug eruption" or "consistent with drug eruption." So, is there a constellation of clinical or histological findings that are diagnostic of drug-induced eruption?

The answer is a qualified yes.

Fixed drug eruption (FDE) and the spectrum of Stevens–Johnson syndrome-toxic epidermal necrolysis (SJS-TEN) are caused almost exclusively by medication.

FDE is quite characteristic, both, clinically and histologically, and is invariably induced by a medication (in spite of the extremely rare observation that food allergy may present clinically and histologically identical to FDE).

The characteristic histological findings in FDE are generally severe dyskeratosis and sometimes complete epidermal necrosis, and a superficial infiltrate of lymphocytes that may also contain eosinophils and/or neutrophils and that may extend into the mid-reticular dermis. In recurrent FDE lesions and sometimes in primary lesions, a large number of melanophages may be admixed in the infiltrate.

Some lesions of FDE, however, are histologically indistinguishable from erythema multiforme; hence, the importance of clinical correlation. Lesions of FDE tend to be fewer and larger than those of EM, randomly rather than symmetrically distributed, and tend to involve mucocutaneous sites such as the lips and external genitalia.

Similarly, cases in the spectrum of *SJS-TEN* are almost invariably caused by medication (*Mycoplasma* is a rare cause of SJS). Histological findings include severe dyskeratosis, often resulting in complete epidermal necrosis; hence, sloughing in the absence of significant infiltrate (rarely an infiltrate often containing eosinophils may be seen). Although highly characteristic, these histological findings are not diagnostic of SJS-TEN. Similar histological findings may be seen in generalized eruptions with sloughing due to other causes, including severe acute photoinduced lupus erythematosus and severe acute graft versus host disease (see Chap. 33), again emphasizing the importance of clinical correlation.

Conclusions

One should avoid using the term "drug eruption" without a morphological descriptor. Drug etiology for an eruption is strongly suspected in cases with extensive keratinocyte dyskeratosis and/or necrosis (FDE, SJS-TEN). In other presentations of medication-induced eruption, histological findings are either unhelpful or at best may raise suspicion for drug etiology. In these cases, confirmation of medication etiology requires further clinical evaluation.

Chapter 10
What Is Pseudolymphoma?

Figure 10.1 illustrates a dense nodular lymphocytic infiltrate.

Nomenclature

Cutaneous lymphoid hyperplasia, reactive lymphoid hyperplasia, lymphocytoma cutis, Spiegler-Fendt sarcoid, pseudolymphoma of Spiegler-Fendt, and lymphadenosis *benigna cutis* are all terms that describe lesions in which there is a dense proliferation of lymphocytes reminiscent of lymphoma but the infiltrate is not malignant. Recently, the term "pseudolymphoma" became widely used for lesions that would have been referred to in the past as one of the other terms.

If There Are No Differences Between the Various Terms, Should We Use One Term Only?

The answer is no. The term lymphocytoma cutis, for example, is best used clinically to describe patients who present with one or less commonly few, red, smooth-fixed nodules on their face. The usefulness of the term pseudolymphoma may be debated.

The term pseudolymphoma is beneficial if used to imply its meaning, namely an infiltrate that on first glance may have been suspected to represent lymphoma but upon further evaluation was proven to be benign by clinical or further histological or molecular evaluation. As such, the adjectival form of pseudolymphoma (pseudolymphomatous) may be more appropriate, as for example in "pseudolymphomatous infiltrate with features characteristic of lymphocytoma cutis" or "pseudolymphomatous infiltrate secondary to tattoo, vaccine, or persistent herpes virus infection…." A clinical and histological attempt to find a cause for a pseudolymphomatous infiltrate should not be overlooked.

The terms Spiegler-Fendt sarcoid, pseudolymphoma of Spiegler-Fendt, and lymphadenosis *benigna cutis*, are old, not specific enough and may be discarded.

D. F. Mutasim, *Practical Skin Pathology*, DOI 10.1007/978-3-319-14729-1_10

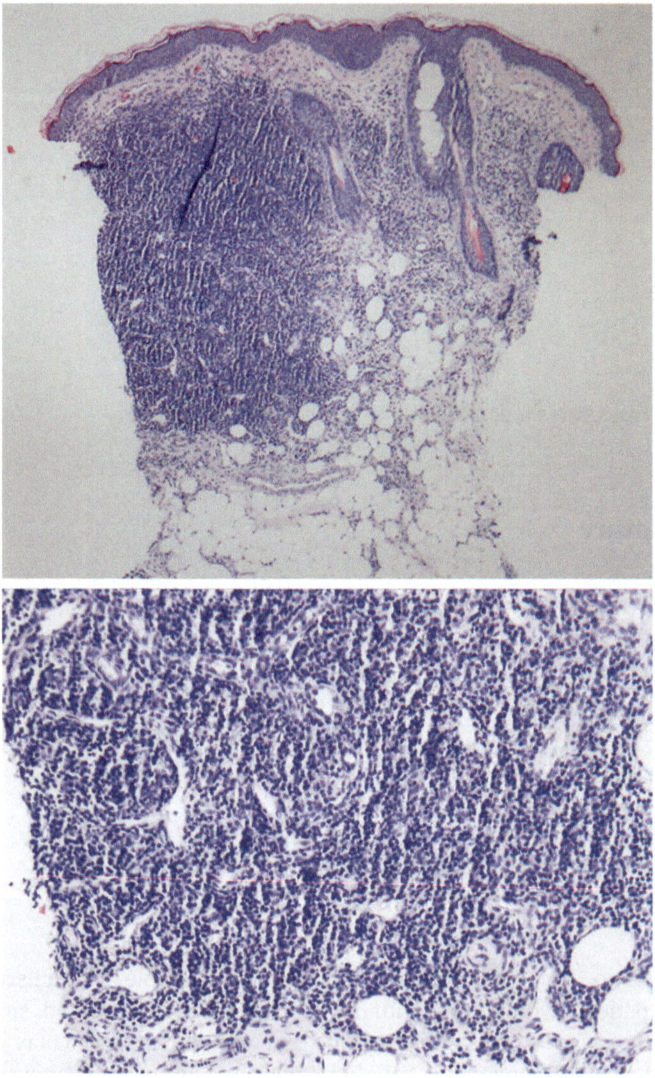

Fig. 10.1 *Top panel* reveals an unremarkable epidermis and papillary dermis. The reticular dermis contains a dense collection of cells. *Bottom panel* reveals a monomorphous infiltrate of small lymphocytes. The biopsy was obtained from a lesion of lymphocytoma cutis on the face

Reactive lymphoid hyperplasia may be appropriate if the inciting agent is identifiable. If not, then the descriptive term cutaneous lymphoid hyperplasia may be the most inclusive, especially that in pathology practice idiopathic cases are the most common, at least in the USA.

What Are Clinical Presentations for This Group of Disorders?

A red, persistent nodule on the face is the most well-known clinical presentation, and is referred to as lymphocytoma cutis. In endemic areas of Europe, this lesion often follows infection with Borrelia. In the USA and other countries, it is idiopathic.

Etiologically identifiable lesions that reveal the histological findings of "pseudolymphoma" occur in nodular scabies (also known as post-scabetic nodules), persistent insect bite reaction (especially to fragments of tick), reaction to tattoo, vaccine, and nodular lesions that may follow healed herpes zoster infection. Close examination of the infiltrate and deeper sections often lead to an accurate diagnosis.

In pathology practice, the commonest provided clinical diagnosis for what turns out to be cutaneous lymphoid hyperplasia is basal cell carcinoma and dermal nevus. The lesion is usually solitary and nondescript.

Conclusions

Just as atypical junctional melanocytic hyperplasia is not a clinical diagnosis but instead a histological description, so is pseudolymphoma. A clinical and histological search for the cause is always required.

Part II
The Clinician's View

Chapter 11
Reddish Facial Papules

Figure 11.1 illustrates two patients with two of the disorders discussed in this chapter.

Case A patient presents with a history of reddish, smooth papules on the face. Some lesions may be follicular and some may be surmounted by a pustule.

Clinical Differential Diagnosis Is

- Rosacea and its variants, steroid rosacea, granulomatous rosacea, periorificial dermatitis, and Demodex folliculitis
- Adult acne
- Bacterial folliculitis
- Pityrosporum folliculitis
- Follicular mucinosis (FM)
- Eosinophilic folliculitis (EF)

Clinical Clues

Acne vulgaris and rosacea and their variants are easily identified by dermatologists; bacterial folliculitis and Pityrosporum folliculitis have extra-facial involvement and are relatively easy to suspect. Both EF and FM may be missed upon initial evaluation.

EF in adults has two clinical presentations with only slight overlap. In one, usually idiopathic, lesions are limited to the face and may be uniformly pustular, hence the term "eosinophilic pustular folliculitis" as reported initially by Ofuji and later in the pediatric literature. In the other, often associated with immune deficiencies including HIV infection, lesions involve the trunk, especially the back. In the setting of HIV infection, lesions are similar to the so-called papular eruption of HIV disease. In both presentations, annular plaques with peripheral pustules may be seen. In some patients, annular plaques with pustules are uniformly seen.

D. F. Mutasim, *Practical Skin Pathology*, DOI 10.1007/978-3-319-14729-1_11

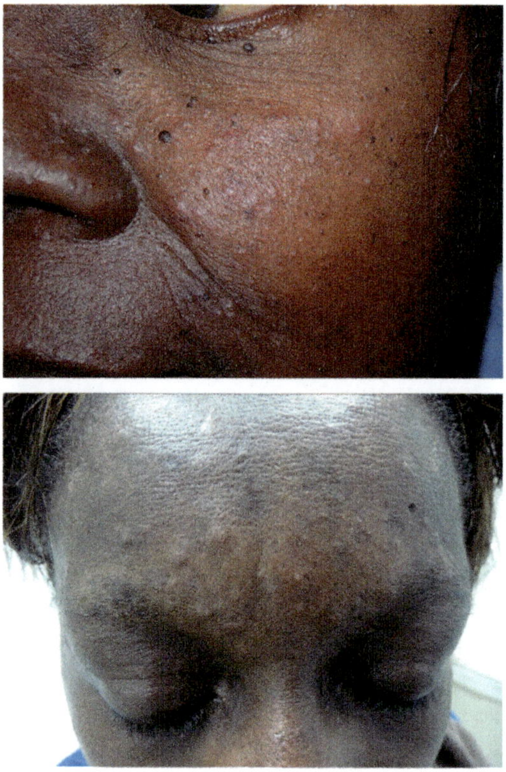

Fig. 11.1 *Upper panel* shows a papular eruption over the face that favors the cheeks. Histological findings are characteristic of granulomatous rosacea. *Lower panel* shows a diffuse papular eruption over the face in a patient with limited scleroderma. Histological examination confirmed eosinophilic folliculitis

FM may be primary or secondary to other cutaneous disorders including mycosis fungoides. Papules of both primary and secondary FM are only faintly reddish, edematous, sometimes boggy, and often confluent into plaques with pea d'orange surface appearance. Lesions in hairy areas are usually alopecic (alopecia mucinosa). Non-facial lesions may be seen in primary and secondary FM, both of which may also have scaly patches or plaques.

How Helpful Is the Pathology?

Very helpful+++

Histological findings

1. *Bacterial* and *pityrosporum folliculitis* are characterized by superficial and or mid follicular neutrophilic abscess.

2. Although *rosacea* is not primarily follicular clinically, the infiltrate involves the follicles often. The presence of neutrophils and/or histiocytes within the infiltrate strongly supports the diagnosis of rosacea. The presence of epithelioid histiocytes and/or multinucleated cells, either in a nodular granulomatous pattern (that may be sarcoidal or tuberculoid) or not, confirms the diagnosis of rosacea and its subtypes in patients presenting with the above clinical findings.

Although none of the above findings is diagnostic of rosacea, the combination of findings usually excludes other suspected diagnoses, hence easily confirming the diagnosis of rosacea. So, regardless of the degree of certainty that the pathologist reports (suggestive of rosacea, consistent with rosacea…) excluding other diagnoses in the above clinical setting can be taken as confirmation of the diagnosis of rosacea.

In other words, the diagnosis of "sarcoidal granuloma" or "tuberculoid granuloma" in a biopsy specimen from a papule on the face in the proper clinical setting is rosacea, unless proven otherwise.

Facial sarcoidosis differs clinically by its color (apple jelly), lack of pustules, and more raised nature of lesions, which may favor mucocutaneous junctions such as eyelids, lips, and nares. Extrafacial lesions are often present.

The differential diagnosis of tuberculoid granuloma in a lesion on the face includes Lupus vulgaris and Leishmania recidivans which are extremely rare except in endemic areas, and is clinically characterized by plaques rather than papules.

So, what is granulomatous rosacea? This term is used by clinical practitioners for a facial eruption with classical features of rosacea plus features of granulomatous inflammation namely an apple jelly appearance, as well as patients with uniformly granulomatous appearing papules in the absence of erythema or telangiectasias. In a rare type of rosacea, acne agminata or acnitis, lesions are characterized by tuberculoid granulomas.

3. *Follicular mucinosis* may involve any part of the skin surface and may be limited to the face, at least in the early stages. The histological diagnosis of follicular mucinosis is rather easy if the biopsy specimen and examined sections contain an involved hair follicle. The presence of follicular spongiosis with mucin confirms the diagnosis. The infiltrate tends to be variable, primarily lymphocytic, and sometimes with eosinophils. This may be missing in small biopsies, superficial biopsies, and due to the loss of the involved follicle during sectioning.

4. Histological differentiation between *eosinophilic folliculitis* and follicular mucinosis may sometimes be difficult. This is especially true if the presence of mucin is slight or questionable and/or the eosinophils are abundant in and around follicular epithelium. In this case, further biopsies would be required. The presence of papulopustules within the eruption and/or the presence of lesions over the trunk strongly favors eosinophilic folliculitis, especially if the patient is immunocompromised.

Therefore, when both follicular mucinosis and eosinophilic folliculitis are within the differential diagnosis of a facial papular eruption, it is suggested that two 3-mm, full-thickness biopsies be obtained. By examining multiple sections of each of the biopsies, the pathologist is highly likely to be able to make the right diagnosis.

Conclusions

In the evaluation of a patient who presents with papules over the face, obtaining two or more biopsy specimens should lead to an accurate diagnosis almost all the time.

Chapter 12
Face infiltrated Plaques/Nodules

Figure 12.1 illustrates two patients with two of the disorders discussed in this chapter.

Case A patient presents with one or few infiltrated facial plaques and/or nodules.
Clinical differential diagnosis consists of

- acute discoid lupus erythematosus (DLE)
- tumid lupus erythematosus TLE
- Jessner benign lymphocytic infiltration of the skin (JBLI)
- lymphocytoma cutis (also known as pseudolymphoma of Spiedler and Fendt)
- sarcoidosis
- granuloma faciale (GF)
- follicular mucinosis and -B-cell lymphoma (BCL).

In endemic areas, lupus vulgaris, Leishmania recidivans, subcutaneous and systemic fungal infection, and extranodal NK-cell lymphoma nasal type may be considered but will not be discussed here.

Clinical Clues

None of the above disorders is symptomatic to any significant degree. Both, sarcoidosis and DLE are seen more commonly among black populations in the USA, but the remaining disorders do not favor race, age, or ethnicity.

Sarcoidosis of the face tends to favor mucocutaneous junctions of the lips, nares, and eyes. The remaining disorders affect various areas of the face equally.

All the above disorders except sarcoidosis and follicular mucinosis strongly favor the face and may be limited to the face.

Lymphocytoma cutis, B-cell lymphoma, and GF are all more likely to present as a solitary lesion.

D. F. Mutasim, *Practical Skin Pathology*, DOI 10.1007/978-3-319-14729-1_12

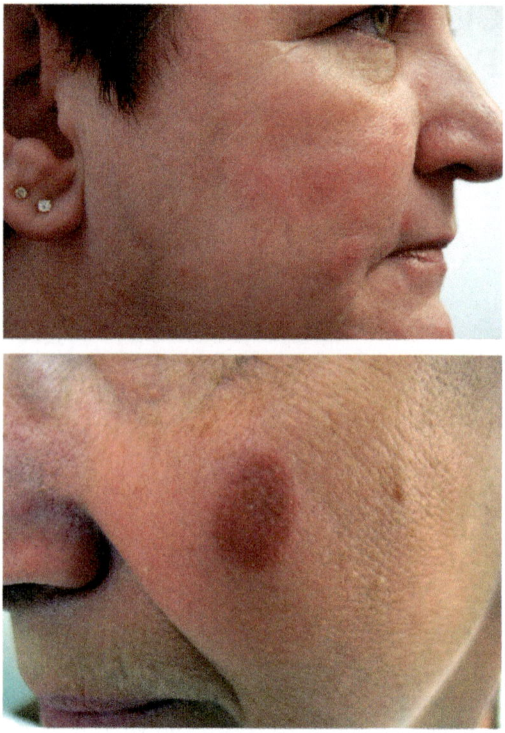

Fig. 12.1 *Upper panel* reveals reddish, smooth edematous plaques over the face. Histological examination revealed primary follicular mucinosis. *Lower panel* reveals a solitary orangish, smooth nodular plaque. Histological examination confirmed the diagnosis of granuloma faciale

Lymphocytoma cutis and B-cell lymphoma present with nodules while DLE, BLI, and follicular mucinosis are more likely to present as plaques. GF and sarcoidosis present as nodules or plaques, and sometimes nodular plaques.

B-cell lymphoma is likely to be a plum-colored nodule or tumor, lymphocytoma cutis a red nodule, GF as an orange nodular plaque, BLI as pink to red plaques and papules, some annular, follicular mucinosis as faintly pink discrete and confluent papules, sarcoidosis as apple jelly papules, and DLE as reddish to purplish plaques with active borders. The surface of all disorders is smooth except an old lesion of DLE, which often acquires both follicular and diffuse scaling.

How Helpful Is the Pathology?

Very helpful +++

Histological Findings

The histological findings in *DLE*, *sarcoidosis*, and *GF* are unique, characteristic, and easily recognizable. There is no debate that chronic DLE and JBLI are different disorders. Differentiation between *tumid LE* and *JBLI* however, may be difficult.

Tumid LE is characterized by minimal or no basal cell vacuolization, with superficial and deep, generally moderate perivascular lymphocytic infiltrate, and variable amounts of interstitial mucin. JBLI is characterized by unremarkable epidermis and a dermal infiltrate that is similar to tumid LE.

Hence, some authors have considered tumid LE and JBLI to be the same disorder. Neither phototesting nor direct immunofluorescence can differentiate between the two disorders with certainty. Patients with both disorders are generally photosensitive. Direct immunofluorescence is generally negative in tumid LE and is negative in JBLI; both disorders respond similarly to treatment.

Some authors have suggested that the two disorders are different but likely related based on multiple common features. Some have suggested that the two disorders should be considered different by virtue of different phenotypic markers of the infiltrating lymphocytes in the two disorders. The heterogeneous immunohistochemical features of the lymphocytes among patients within each disorder, however, make the above conclusion unconvincing.

Yet, others have suggested that BLI represents a benign lymphocytic proliferation that may be viewed as a perivascular form of lymphocytoma cutis. It is highly likely that a biopsy specimen may be interpreted by one pathologist as representing JBLI and by another as tumid LE, based on their training and views. For the clinician, it may be worth accepting this difficulty and uncertainty. The majority of patients with tumid LE do not have internal organ involvement (of SLE), and are treated similarly to patients with JBLI.

Alternatively, the clinician may choose to give the diagnosis of JPLI to patients with predominant or exclusive facial involvement, especially if the number of lesions was few and some were annular (as Jessner and Kanof described in their patients), while the diagnosis of tumid LE be given to those with predominant extra facial involvement.

Follicular mucinosis may be an isolated disorder, so-called primary follicular mucinosis (also referred to as alopecia mucinosa) or secondary to mycosis fungoides (MF). It is important to note here that mucin deposition within follicular epithelium may be seen in several inflammatory and neoplastic dermatological disorders, where it is viewed as a coincidental finding.

Primary follicular mucinosis reveals a perivascular and perifollicular lymphocytic infiltrate with or without eosinophils with exocytosis and spongiosis, and mucin deposition in follicular epithelium. In MF-associated follicular mucinosis, histological findings of mycosis fungoides are also present, namely single or grouped lymphocytes with halos in the epidermis.

Clonal proliferation of T-lymphocytes is documented, by gene rearrangement studies, in MF-associated follicular mucinosis and only rarely in primary follicular mucinosis. Follicular mucinosis in younger individuals is likely to be the primary disorder while older patients are much more likely to have MF-associated follicular mucinosis.

Lymphocytoma cutis is characterized histologically by one or few superficial nodular collections of small lymphocytes, with or without germinal centers. (Refer to Chap. 11, Sect. 11.2, on pseudolymphoma.)

B-cell lymphoma involving the face is most likely follicle center cell type, and may present histologically with a nodular and or diffuse lymphocytic infiltrate, that is, more intense and deeper than the infiltrate in lymphocytoma cutis and other pseudolymphomas. In questionable cases, immunohistochemical and molecular genetic studies for clonality may be needed.

Conclusions

In the evaluation of patients with plaques and/or nodules over the face, histological examination is extremely helpful and often essential.

Chapter 13
Patchy Alopecia

Figure 13.1 illustrates two patients with two of the disorders discussed in this chapter.

Case A patient presents with multiple patches of complete alopecia over the scalp.

Clinical differential diagnosis is well known to dermatologists and is divided between so-called nonscarring and scarring alopecia. As the term "scarring" refers to a specific type of dermal fibrosis, which lacks in most disorders referred to as scarring alopecia, a better term may be irreversible or permanent patchy alopecia. Reversible or nonpermanent patchy alopecia in almost all cases is *alopecia areata*. Permanent patchy alopecia is most often

- lichen planopilaris, LPP and less frequently
- DLE
- pseudopelade, and
- folliculitis decalvans.

Clinical Clues

Alopecia areata is easily recognizable by its history of rather acute onset, early age of onset, randomly scattered patches, no loss of the follicular ostia, presence of exclamation hairs, frequent spontaneous regrowth of hair, and the occasional presence of patches of hair loss over the face.

LPP tends to favor middle-aged women and has an insidious onset; hence, patients present to a dermatologist several months after the onset of hair loss. It also strongly favors the vertex and crown of the scalp, may be rarely associated with other manifestations of lichen planus including genital lesions and facial papules, and upon examination, reveals the characteristic "footsteps in the snow" appearance of generally 1–1.5 cm round to oval patches of invariably complete alopecia, surrounded by a narrow rim of activity consisting of pinpoint-to-1 mm, pinkish to violaceous papules made up of keratin in the follicular ostium. The combination of these findings is so characteristic that a biopsy may not be required.

D. F. Mutasim, *Practical Skin Pathology*, DOI 10.1007/978-3-319-14729-1_13

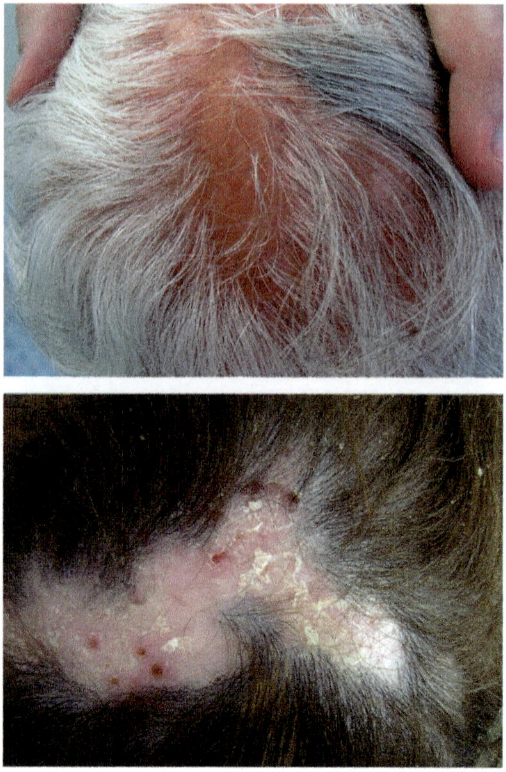

Fig. 13.1 *Upper panel* reveals centrally confluent hairless smooth patches, characteristic of lichen planopilaris. *Lower panel* reveals closely set hairless patches with scaling and excoriations in a patient with discoid lupus erythematosus

DLE may cause smooth patches of cicatricial alopecia only rarely. I have seen around 200 patients with DLE, among whom only one had smooth patches of hair loss limited to the scalp and with a smooth surface. In general, the surface of lesions of DLE is scaly, often with follicular keratotic plugging, and diffuse erythema in addition to induration, especially at the borders. To my surprise, in the patient referred to above, the histological findings of more than one biopsy specimen did reveal basal vacuolization and a superficial and deep lymphocytic infiltrate with mucin characteristic of acute DLE. The other epidermal findings of DLE were all absent; hence, contributing to the smooth surface of lesions.

Pseudopelade is a historical term, which was initially coined to describe a disorder that looked grossly like alopecia areata but, in which, hair loss was permanent and irreversible. As per the initial description, especially in the last three decades, the nosology of pseudopelade has been debated extensively.

Some adhere to the view that pseudopelade is a clinical descriptive term rather than a true disorder, and that the term should apply to end-stage patchy permanent alopecia whether it results from LPP, DLE, folliculitis decalvans, or other disorders. In this view, the term may be deleted from the dermatology lexicon or used in cases for which the exact etiology of patchy cicatricial alopecia is not known at the time.

Others subscribe to the view that pseudopelade is a primary disorder whose end-stage is patchy permanent alopecia but may be identified in the early stages by continued activity (progression of alopecia) in the absence of characteristic clinical findings of LPP. Those who subscribe to the first view respond to this claim by suggesting that the lack of clinical evidence of LPP does not exclude the diagnosis especially in view of the fact that evidence of mild clinical activity in LPP may be missed or missing. The evidence presented for this argument is the observation that clinically inactive border of complete alopecia patches may still reveal histological evidence of inflammation as in active cases of LPP.

In my early years of practice, I subscribed to the second view that pseudopelade is a primary disorder. Having seen and managed around 40 patients and evaluated histologically dozens of biopsies, I believe the only reason to retain the term "pseudopelade" is historical, in honor of Dr. Brocq, who contributed extensively to clinical dermatology. The disorder behind every patient with patches of permanent alopecia should be sought after. Only when a patient presents at the end-stage of the disorder with no characteristic features should the term be used, only because it appears more medical than patchy cicatricial alopecia and gives the patient a name for the disorder.

Folliculitis Decalvans is an inflammatory disorder of the superficial portion of hair follicles almost exclusively seen in African-American men. Patches of complete alopecia are surrounded by follicular pustules. Patches enlarge as pustules involute, resulting in further loss of hair. Some involved hair follicles have multiple hair shafts within their ostia. Some patients, including Caucasians, do not have the classical presentation of folliculitis decalvans, but instead have a progressive follicular scarring process of the scalp with predominance of tufted follicles. These patients have been referred to as having "tufted folliculitis." Whether tufted folliculitis is a primary disorder or a variant of folliculitis decalvans may be debated.

Rare causes of patchy alopecia of the scalp include secondary syphilis, sarcoidosis, and metastatic disease all associated with other historical and clinical findings that help make the diagnosis. One patch of permanent alopecia on the temporal scalp since a young age is likely triangular alopecia.

How Helpful Is the Pathology?

Very helpful+++

Histological Clues

For a scalp biopsy specimen to be adequate for histological evaluation, it should be at least 4 mm and contain abundant fat. Transverse sections are generally superior to longitudinal sections by allowing examination of all follicular units at various depths. Some have proposed that two biopsy specimens be obtained; one for transverse sectioning and the other for longitudinal sectioning. If one biopsy specimen is obtained, it is preferable that it be sectioned transversely.

Lesions of active *DLE* are so characteristic clinically (and histologically) that the need for a biopsy is questionable. Because of the general seriousness of the disorder, most dermatologists do obtain a biopsy to confirm their clinical impression. The characteristic histological findings of DLE are easily recognizable, albeit variable: parakeratosis, epidermal atrophy, basal vacuolization, dilated hair follicles that may contain compact keratin, dilated capillaries admixed with melanophages, and a superficial and deep lymphocytic infiltrate around blood vessels adjacent to follicular epithelium, and very rarely hugging the follicular epithelium (the latter being a feature of LPP). Interstitial mucin deposition may also be present. Late lesions may reveal dermal fibrosis.

The above picture is seen in the majority of DLE cases. Occasionally, DLE may present differently. The infiltrate in DLE may also be lichenoid along the folliculo–dermal or the dermo–epidermal junction, bringing up the possibility of overlap with LPP (in the former), or overlap with LP (in the latter) as in lichenoid lupus or LP/LE overlap, two names that some believe may represent one disorder.

Rarely instead of epidermal atrophy, one may find epidermal hyperplasia, sometimes along with papillomatosis (so-called hypertrophic DLE). If the biopsy specimen is superficial, the diagnosis may be missed for disorders with primary epidermal hyperplasia. Direct immunofluorescence in this case is usually diagnostic (immunoglobulins and complement along the dermo–epidermal junction). Rarely, neither basal vacuolization is present nor are there superficial melanophages to suggest its occurrence earlier. In such cases, the clinical appearance of lesions is that of tumid LE.

Biopsy specimens from the active border of lesions of *LPP* also reveal characteristic findings: a rather dense lymphocytic infiltrate that hugs the superficial portion of the hair follicle (which is often surrounded by a prominent fibro–mucinous sheath), resulting in obscuring of follicular basal cells, just as the infiltrate in LP obscures the basal cells at the dermo–epidermal junction. The follicular infundibulum may be dilated and often contains excessive keratin. Rarely are lesions of LPP accompanied by interfollicular epidermal findings of LP.

So what about *pseudopelade*?

As per the above discussion, pseudopelade is best not used as a specific diagnosis but synonymous with end-stage irreversible (cicatricial) alopecia. A cause should be pursued by obtaining further biopsies for histological and immunofluorescence examination, taking history into consideration and making the best clinicopathological correlation possible.

Pustules of *folliculitis decalvans* and tufted folliculitis reveal a neutrophilic abscess early on followed by histiocytes and multinucleated cells that strongly favors the superficial portion of the hair follicle. Older lesions reveal scar fibrosis and loss of hair follicles.

Conclusions

In a patient presenting with patches of alopecia, one should first determine whether follicular ostia are present, which strongly suggests that hair follicles are still present or whether they are absent. If in doubt or follicular ostia are not present then at least one biopsy specimen from the border of alopecic patches should be obtained. By far, the most likely diagnosis would be LPP. If the diagnosis of LPP, however, is not confirmed, then further biopsies or a search for another diagnosis should be pursued. The use of the term “pseudopelade” as a primary disorder should be discouraged.

Chapter 14
Diffuse Smooth Alopecia

Figure 14.1 illustrates two patients with two of the disorders discussed in this chapter.

Case A 55-year-old white woman presents with the complaint "I am losing my hair," or "my hair is thinning," or "my hairdresser told me that I'm losing my hair."

These and other similar statements are commonly heard by dermatologists and often cause a slight state anxiety. Questions that often arise in the mind of the dermatologist include:

- Will the physical findings be diagnostic?
- Will I need to do a biopsy,
- Will I have to do hormonal and systemic evaluation?
- Will the patient have one disorder or more?
- Will I be able to help the patient?

In this presentation, physical examination and histological findings may be only moderately helpful. History, especially, if provided accurately by the patient, is extremely helpful and is able to put the patient in one of two major categories of hair loss.

History

Increased hair shedding is characteristic of diffuse alopecia areata AA and telogen effluvium TE. Patients with TE and AA either volunteer or respond to questioning by admitting that they are "losing hair" or "shedding more hair than usual" for a definable period of time.

On the other hand, patients with hair loss secondary to androgenetic alopecia, systemic causes, or drugs report progressive hair thinning over a longer period of time of several months to a few years that may be brought to their attention by a hairdresser, friend, or relative.

D. F. Mutasim, *Practical Skin Pathology*, DOI 10.1007/978-3-319-14729-1_14

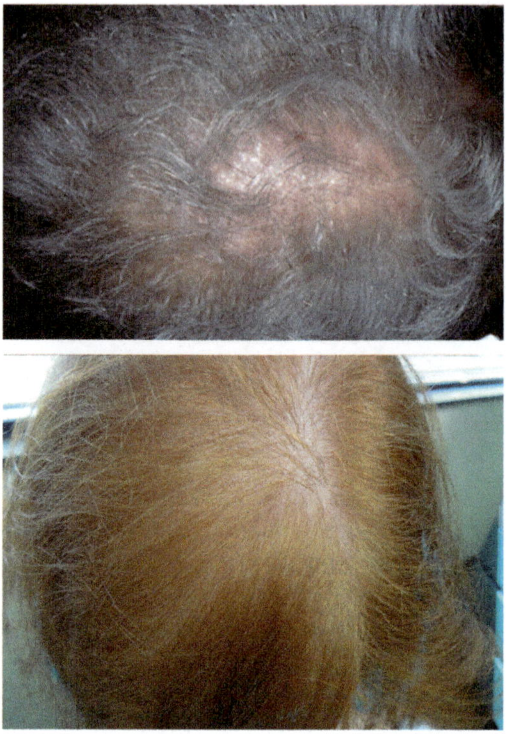

Fig. 14.1 *Upper panel* reveals a middle-aged woman with severe diffuse alopecia secondary to telogen effluvium. *Lower panel* reveals an 18-year-old woman with severe early onset androgenetic alopecia

Further questioning includes:

- Hormonal status (menopause, hormone replacement, and history of surgical removal of the ovaries)
- List of medications and their duration
- History of recent febrile illness, surgery, and other traumatic experiences
- Family history of scalp hair thinning in siblings and both parents
- Detailed medical history
- Hair styling techniques (more applicable in African–American women)

Physical Examination

Physical examination of the scalp is aimed at determining the following:

- Presence of skin surface findings such as erythema and scaling (this chapter presupposes that the scalp appearance is normal)
- Confirming that the hair loss is diffuse, rather than patchy (patchy hair loss is discussed in Chap. 13)
- Assessing the degree of hair loss with the realization that if hair thinning can be appreciated by simple inspection, then hair loss is significant
- Assessing the predominant sites of involvement, specifically, whether the hair loss is diffuse or favors the top or vertex of the scalp

- Assessing the degree of telogen shift (characteristic of both active AA and active TE) by a gentle hair pull test
- Looking for signs of hyperandrogenization such as hirsutism and acne
- Looking for signs of alopecia areata involving other hairy areas such as the axilla and pubic area
- Looking for skin signs of systemic disease, such as iron deficiency and hyper- or hypothyroidism, which are well known to dermatologists.

How Helpful Is the Pathology?

Moderately ++

The Scalp Biopsy

It is recommended that two biopsy specimens are obtained for the evaluation of patients with diffuse alopecia. Sections from one specimen are to be obtained longitudinally and the other transversely. Some pathologists (including the author) choose to section both specimens transversely. If one biopsy specimen is submitted, most pathologists elect to obtain transverse sections. Although the processing and interpretation of transverse sections is more laborious, they provide valuable information that may not be obtained by longitudinal sections. Transverse sections sample all the hair follicles in the specimen at all levels, while a longitudinal section samples four or five only. The multiple segments of the hair follicle throughout its entirety are more easily visualized in transverse sections.

In obtaining a scalp biopsy specimen for the evaluation of alopecia, it is important that subcutaneous fat is included in order to visualize the bulbs of terminal hairs. It is suggested that the clinician who obtains only one biopsy specimen indicate it on the requisition form for the pathologist to obtain transverse sections in case the specimen got sectioned longitudinally due to oversight by the pathology technician.

Histological Findings

The histological findings of diffuse AA, TE, and androgenetic alopecia are highly characteristic. They are also highly dynamic, that is, they change with time, which adds a degree of difficulty to their interpretation. Occasionally, one may not be able to make a specific diagnosis. Finally, there is some degree of overlap between the findings of AA and TE depending on the stage of the disorder.

In order to understand the histological findings in the above disorders, it is important to recall the normal dynamic cycling of the hair follicle. On the scalp, approximately 10% of the terminal hair follicles are in the resting catagen/telogen phase and the rest are in the growing anagen phase. In *androgenetic alopecia*, there is a shift from terminal to vellus hairs. Terminal hairs undergo progressive miniaturization over a few, shortened, hair cycles and become clinically invisible; hence, hair thinning or alopecia. Unlike scalp terminal hairs whose bulbs reside in the subcutaneous fat, vellus hair follicles reside in the superficial reticular dermis similar to those on the face (except the male beard area). In long-standing androgenetic alopecia, hair follicles may involute completely. The progressive miniaturization of hair follicles is driven by androgens. Many biopsies of androgenetic alopecia have a mild perivascular lymphocytic infiltrate in the superficial dermis but its significance is not known yet. Miniaturization in androgenetic alopecia is not associated with fibrosis or scarring.

The predominant sites of involvement in androgenetic alopecia are well known in men and women. For obvious reasons, the vast majority of biopsy specimens obtained to exclude or confirm androgenetic alopecia are from women.

In diffuse AA (which is extremely rare when compared to classic AA), an inflammatory response that is likely autoimmune in origin surrounds the anagen hair bulb resulting in accelerated regression to catagen/telogen. This is followed by shedding of the hair, leading to hair loss. The histological findings of *diffuse AA* are similar to those of classic patchy AA; namely a lymphocytic infiltrate surrounding the hair bulb and appearing as “a swarm of bees” hugging the bulb. The duration of the infiltrate varies. The activity may subside either spontaneously or with treatment, and the hair regression is reversed back to normal.

In patients with *TE*, there is a similar shift or regression of anagen hairs to telogen hairs. Unlike AA, this regression follows a significant systemic event such as delivery, high fever, long surgery, severe, rapid weight loss, and the like. Its mechanism is not well understood. A few weeks to a few months following the causative event, many hairs that have regressed to telogen start shedding. Like diffuse AA, hair shedding in TE is diffuse.

A biopsy specimen obtained in the early or active phase of TE reveals a significant anagen to catagen/telogen shift. Compared to scalp anagen hair follicles, telogen hair follicles are smaller and regress outwardly, that is, their epithelium is seen in the mid- to superficial reticular dermis. Unlike active lesions of diffuse AA, there is no infiltrate in lesions of TE. Transverse sections of the lowest one third of a biopsy of TE consisting of fat may have very few hair follicles. The mid- and superficial portions of the specimen, however, reveal a normal complement of hair follicles, a large percentage of which are in catagen/telogen.

Biopsy specimens of diffuse hair thinning secondary to *systemic disorder or drug* are not specific and their diagnosis is made by exclusion.

Limitations in the Interpretation of Scalp Biopsy Specimens

There are a few reasons that make coming up with an accurate and specific diagnosis in all scalp biopsy specimens not possible.

1. Disorders may overlap.

This is particularly true of TE and androgenetic alopecia. Some women present with definite history of increased hair shedding, yet examination yields findings of androgenetic alopecia, such as widening of the parting of hair or diffuse hair thinning favoring the crown and sparing the frontal hairline, characteristic of female-pattern alopecia. At least, some of these patients turn out to have a baseline of androgenetic alopecia that has been overlooked by the patient or hairdresser due to its insidious onset and slow progression. The superimposition of hair shedding due to TE brings the patient to the dermatologist.

2. TE and diffuse AA may be histologically difficult to differentiate.

Both groups of patients report increased recent hair shedding. Like patients with TE, some patients with diffuse AA also relate the onset of their disorder to a recent event. The hairs which are pulled out easily in both disorders are club telogen hairs. Exclamation hairs may not be as easily seen in diffuse AA as in patchy AA. As mentioned earlier, the histological findings in AA and TE may overlap, depending on the stage of disease when the biopsy was obtained. Both disorders show an increased telogen to anagen ratio, and differ in the presence of lymphocytes surrounding hair bulbs in active AA.

3. Alopecia secondary to medication or systemic disorder does not reveal characteristic histological findings; hence, its diagnosis is firmly based on clinical and laboratory evaluation (pathologists rarely receive biopsy specimens to confirm or exclude hair thinning secondary to medication or systemic disorder).

Conclusions

In the evaluation of a woman with diffuse hair thinning, a detailed history is essential. By adding the physical findings, an accurate diagnosis may be reached in a large number of patients. A biopsy specimen may be performed in order to confirm a clinical diagnosis or in search for a diagnosis. Providing information about history and clinical findings to the pathologist is helpful.

Chapter 15
Follicular Pustules of the Scalp

Figure 15.1 illustrates two patients with two of the disorders discussed in this chapter.

Case A patient presents with recurrent lesions over the scalp that start as pustules. Examination reveals crusted excoriations and a rare follicular papule or pustule. Few small hairless patches are also present. The remainder of skin examination is unremarkable.

Clinical differential diagnosis includes

- bacterial folliculitis
- folliculitis decalvans
- erosive pustular dermatosis EPD
- fungal folliculitis, and
- acne necrotica.

Clinical Clues

Patients with *bacterial folliculitis* of the scalp frequently excoriate the lesions, so physical examination may not reveal intact pustules, making the diagnosis often difficult. In addition, patients with scalp pruritus may develop secondary bacterial folliculitis due to scratching. Determining whether the bacterial folliculitis is primary or secondary may be difficult. A therapeutic trial with antibiotics is justifiable in such cases. If intact pustules are present, bacterial cultures should be obtained.

In adults, *fungal folliculitis* (tinea capitis) is extremely rare. Clues to its diagnosis include breakage of hair close to the scalp and sometimes scaling. In adults, a kerion may be misdiagnosed as dissecting cellulitis. A high index of suspicion is required in order to make the diagnosis. Pityrosporum folliculitis involves the trunk most commonly, the face occasionally, and the scalp rarely.

Folliculitis decalvans is almost limited to adult black men. The author has seen only one woman and two non-black men with the disorder. Unlike lesions of bacterial folliculitis of the scalp, pustules are most likely to be seen in patients with

D. F. Mutasim, *Practical Skin Pathology*, DOI 10.1007/978-3-319-14729-1_15

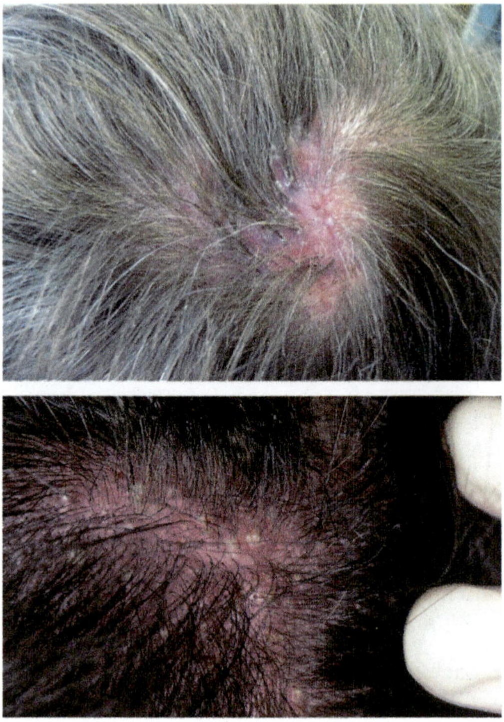

Fig. 15.1 *Upper panel* demonstrates partial hair loss with underlying erythema and tufts of hair in tufted folliculitis. *Lower panel* demonstrates a Caucasian patient with sterile follicular pustules and mild hair loss; variant of folliculitis decalvans

folliculitis decalvans, especially at the border of patches of scarring alopecia. In the early stages, however, the diagnosis may be difficult to make in the absence of patches of scarring alopecia. The impression of footsteps in the snow with surrounding pustules is easily recognized by dermatologists as folliculitis decalvans.

EPD is a scalp disorder that favors the elderly and that is often reported to follow trauma. Patients present with both individual pustules as well as "lakes of pus" either beneath a layer of keratin or matted with hair. The etiology of EPD is not known. The disorder responds dramatically to topical steroids.

Occasionally, patients with active *lichen planopilaris* may develop a pustule at the site of an involved hair follicle at the border of a patch of alopecia. In general, however, pustules are rare, secondary, and very few in number compared to follicular scaly papules. In addition, lichen planopilaris most commonly affects middle-aged women, and is rare in young black men.

Acne necrotica is a rare disorder that favors men. The primary lesion, a follicular papule or pustule, is rarely seen; in its place (which is the site where patients point to) a scar is present. The lesions usually number in the few and are limited to the scalp. Although acne necrotica shares some clinical features with acnitis of the face, there is no evidence that the two disorders are related.

A rare patient with *dermatitis herpetiformis* (DH) may have predominant (posterior) scalp involvement with vesiculo-pustules, and may not be aware of minor involvement elsewhere. The diagnosis of DH should be suspected if the patient does not respond to folliculitis treatment or the lesions favor the posterior aspect of the scalp with possible extension to the posterior neck. Examination of other commonly affected body sites, such as elbows, knees, and buttocks, is likely to reveal few active or healing lesions.

How Helpful Is the Pathology?

Not much +

Histological Clues

Patients with the above disorders often do not have a primary lesion to examine or to obtain a biopsy specimen. History, prior response to treatments, and comprehensive skin examination are often all that the dermatologist has at her/his disposal. A biopsy specimen is not always required if clinical suspicion is strong and/or response to treatment is satisfactory. Cultures for organisms may be helpful and therapeutic trials necessary.

If an intact pustule is found and biopsied, the histological findings are invariably a neutrophilic pustule in the superficial portion of a hair follicle consistent with both infectious and noninfectious folliculitis. Microbial organisms may be present. The primary lesion of acne necrotica is that of lymphocytic folliculitis and perifolliculitis, and the primary lesion in dermatitis herpetiformis consists of a collection of neutrophils in the papillary dermis.

Conclusions

In the evaluation of patients with history of follicular papules and/or pustules of the scalp, history and examination as well as responses to treatments often yield more information than histopathology.

Chapter 16
Scaly Scalp

Figure 16.1 illustrates two patients with two of the disorders discussed in this chapter.

Case A patient presents with scaly scalp.

Differential Diagnosis includes four common disorders

- pityriasis capitis (known as dandruff and in the distant past as "seborrhea sicca")
- seborrheic dermatitis
- psoriasis, and
- tinea capitis'

two rare disorders

- dermatomyositis and
- acute Langerhan cell histiocytosis

and two disorders that are not definitively distinct but instead are morphological descriptive terms

- sebopsoriasis and
- tinea amiantacea

Clinical Clues *Dandruff* or pityriasis capitis is among the most common skin disorders and is easily recognized by a dry, flaky scalp. The disorder has been thought to be due to abnormality in sebaceous glands for over a century, hence the old term "seborrhea sicca," and should be distinguished from seborrheic dermatitis, a related disorder but with oily or greasy scaling. Both disorders may be pruritic and are believed to be due to infection with *Malassezia*. Both respond to the same treatment, which is why patients with dandruff are labeled by dermatologists as having seborrheic dermatitis. Younger generations of dermatologists may not even recognize dandruff as a separate disorder from seborrheic dermatitis.

Dandruff consists of generally diffuse, fine, dry, flaky scaling, while *seborrheic dermatitis* reveals mild erythema and glistening greasy scale. Although dandruff is

D. F. Mutasim, *Practical Skin Pathology*, DOI 10.1007/978-3-319-14729-1_16

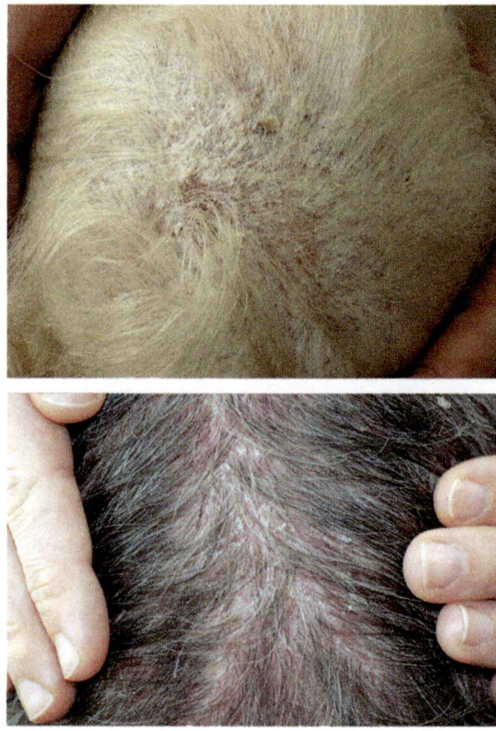

Fig. 16.1 *Upper panel* demonstrates an older woman with diffuse, whitish scaling of her scalp secondary to erythrodermic psoriasis. *Lower panel* demonstrates mild erythema and diffuse scaling secondary to pemphigus foliaceous that may be confused for scaly scalp. Closer inspection revealed superficial erosions beneath the keratinaceous material

a phenomenon of the scalp, seborrheic dermatitis may involve multiple sites over the face, ears, anogenital skin, mid-chest, mid-back, and skin folds. It is easiest to recognize over the face. When it involves skin folds, it may be mistaken for intertrigo.

Face lesions in dark-skinned individuals, especially African-Americans, may be annular and be confused for other disorders, including sarcoidosis and discoid lupus erythematosus (DLE).

Psoriasis of the scalp is generally in the form of individual plaques but may be diffuse. In general, the scale is thicker and whiter, and the lateral margin of the plaques is brightly red. Facial psoriasis in patients with scalp psoriasis is extremely rare compared to facial involvement in patients with scalp seborrheic dermatitis. External ear involvement may be seen in both disorders. Limited plaque psoriasis elsewhere should be sought after and its presence is usually helpful in difficult cases.

The exact meaning of *sebopsoriasis* is not clear. There are no clinical criteria for the diagnosis of sebopsoriasis. A literature search produced a little over 400 references to sebopsoriasis. Some authors use the term to refer to seborrheic dermatitis in patients with psoriasis with the view that it is seborrheic dermatitis that has acquired psoriasis like features due to the Koebner phenomenon. Others use the term to refer to psoriasis in seborrheic areas with special reference to the face. Yet others classify facial psoriasis into three subtypes, namely, hairline psoriasis (an extension of scalp psoriasis), "true" psoriasis, and sebopsoriasis. Those who use the term, agree that the morphology of lesions of sebopsoriasis is intermediate between psoriasis and seborrheic dermatitis.

Two important questions that do not have clear answers are whether sebopsoriasis exists as the sole presentation of psoriasis; and, whether it may be limited to the scalp.

In practice, some dermatologists use the term sebopsoriasis for scaling of the scalp that is not characteristic of either seborrheic dermatitis or psoriasis, but instead is intermediate between the two. It is well known that the histological findings of seborrheic dermatitis mimic those of psoriasis; hence, in these patients histopathology is most frequently not helpful and is often interpreted as psoriasiform dermatitis consistent with both disorders.

There is some evidence that sebopsoriasis, like seborrheic dermatitis, is caused by *Malassezia* organisms and responds to the same treatment, making differentiation between the two disorders as the cause of a scaly scalp of little practical value.

Tinea capitis as a cause of diffusely scaly scalp is almost limited to children and is extremely rare in adults. Features that should raise suspicion for a fungal infection include follicular papules or follicular pustules as well as broken hairs. If microscopic examination of hairs does not confirm the presence of fungal organisms, culture and/or histological examination of a biopsy specimen may be required.

Tinea amiantacea was described many decades ago. Patients are children who present with tightly adherent, thick, whitish keratinous material at the base of the hairs. Attempts at removing the material are difficult and often result in removing some hairs. Admixture of crust may sometimes be seen. The underlying scalp may be erythematous, dry, or wet. The etiology of tinea amiantacea is not known. Whether the condition is a primary disorder or a manifestation of other disorders of the scalp has been debated. Most evidence indicates that it may be an unusual manifestation of psoriasis, atopic dermatitis, or seborrheic dermatitis. In attempting to make a specific diagnosis, one disease may be favored over the others if the patient has manifestations of it elsewhere on the skin or has strong family history.

Adult-onset presentation of what appears as tinea amiantacea may represent pemphigus vulgaris or pemphigus foliaceous. I have seen few patients who were treated for scalp psoriasis and or tinea capitis for many months before a biopsy was performed and confirmed pemphigus.

In infants and young children, scalp lesions that are clinically very similar to seborrheic dermatitis may be a manifestation of *Langerhans cell histiocytosis* especially if the lesions are purpuric. Most patients have lesions elsewhere and are frequently sick with failure to thrive and organomegaly.

Finally, scalp lesions of *dermatomyositis* may be confused for other disorders, especially if the manifestations of dermatomyositis elsewhere are not obvious or the patient did not bring up the other lesions to the attention of the dermatologist. Scalp lesions in dermatomyositis are often diffuse. In addition to the fine whitish scaling, lesions are erythematous, atrophic, with telangiectasias, and are markedly pruritic. In my experience of 50–60 patients, more than 90 % of the patients with dermatomyositis have scalp involvement, and most of them are highly symptomatic.

How Helpful Is the Pathology?

Moderately ++

Histological Findings

Biopsies are rarely obtained in patients with scaly scalp. Clinical diagnosis is often adequate. Histopathology may be helpful in confirming dermatomyositis, tinea capitis, and Langerhan cell histiocytosis. In clinically difficult cases, histological differentiation among seborrheic dermatitis, sebopsoriasis, and psoriasis is not satisfactory. A biopsy often reveals a combination of psoriasiform epidermal hyperplasia, spongiosis, and neutrophils and serum in the parakeratosis.

Conclusions

In the evaluation of patients with scaly scalp, the attempt at making a clinical diagnosis is often satisfactory. For patients who do not respond to the treatment, histological evaluation may be required.

Chapter 17
Oral Erosions

Figure 17.1 illustrates two patients with two of the disorders discussed in this chapter.

Case A patient presents with several-month history of painful oral erosions. Examination reveals erosions (not ulcers), involving any combination of the buccal mucosa, gingiva, tongue, and lips. Symptoms suggesting pharyngeal and/or laryngeal and/or esophageal involvement could be present.

Clinical Differential Diagnosis The differential diagnosis includes

- *erosive lichen planus* (LP)
- *mucosal pemphigoid* (MP) and
- *pemphigus vulgaris* (*PV*).

In case of acute onset strong consideration would be given to oral or mucosal erythema multiforme; hand, foot, and mouth disease, and other rare viral and bacterial oral infections. If the lesions are ulcers, then aphthosis is the preferred diagnosis.

Clinical Clues The likelihood of making the right diagnosis solely based on clinical findings is at best moderate. Vesicles may rarely be seen in all three disorders. The degree of pain is probably worst in patients with PV, but cannot be relied upon in the clinical evaluation of patients.

Both erosive LP and PV favor the buccal mucosa. PV may be limited to the buccal mucosa, especially the posterior part. Erosive LP may be limited to the buccal mucosa, often favoring the anterior portion and occasionally extending to the corner of the mouth and lips.

Although MP has also traditionally been referred to as cicatricial pemphigoid because of the tendency for scarring, several patients with oral MP do not have evidence of scarring, so the diagnosis should be considered in the absence of scarring. Similarly, although erosive LP may be associated with striated whitish patches involving the surrounding mucosa, some patients with erosive LP have erosions without the characteristic surrounding whitish striations.

In my experience, patients with oral erosive LP are much more likely than PV, and MP to have genital involvement as well. Concomitant ocular involvement is

D. F. Mutasim, *Practical Skin Pathology*, DOI 10.1007/978-3-319-14729-1_17

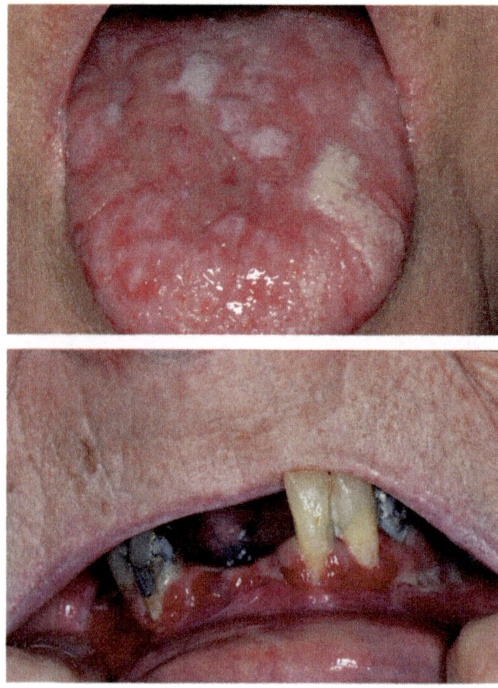

Fig. 17.1 *Upper panel* demonstrates extensive superficial ulcers over the tongue in an elderly woman with severe oral lichen planus and limited skin lesions. *Lower panel* demonstrates diffuse gingival erosions in a patient with oral and cutaneous pemphigoid

almost diagnostic of MP; LP involves the eyes very rarely and PV almost never. PV is more likely to have an overlooked scalp or facial lesion, and rarely a lesion of the upper trunk. Both PV and MP are more likely to have lesions extend to the pharynx and/or larynx.

The clinical presentation of inflammation and desquamation of the gingiva, referred to as *desquamative gingivitis*, is most often a manifestation of LP and to a slightly lesser extent MP and only rarely PV. Of around 100 patients with PV that I have seen, (almost all with oral lesions), only one had lesions limited to the gingiva.

How Helpful Is the Pathology?

Very helpful +++

Histopathology and Immunofluorescence

Because of the potentially serious implications of the above disorders and differences in treatment, biopsy evaluation is essential. It is important to evaluate both histopathology and immunofluorescence. Except if the lesions are limited to the palate or gingiva, a dermatologist is highly qualified to perform an oral mucosal biopsy. Mucosal epithelium is forgiving and sutures are not always necessary. In order to perform biopsy on the less accessible posterior buccal mucosa, a suture may be placed at the site of the intended biopsy and the mucosa pulled out. Sharp scissors or a no. 15 blade on a handle may then be used to obtain the pulled tissue. Pressure is then applied to the site for homeostasis or a suture may be placed. Palate or gingival biopsies are better obtained by an oral surgeon.

The specimen for histological evaluation should include the border of the erosion along with adjacent, usually inflamed epithelium while the biopsy for immunofluorescence should be obtained from normal-appearing mucosa just beyond the site of inflammation. In patients with desquamative gingivitis, a surgical biopsy may be substituted by an epithelial sheet. A sheet may be obtained by the patient dislodging it by rolling their tongue along with a slight suctioning force and placing it in the appropriate bottle for histology and immunofluorescence. Evaluation of both specimens in concert leads to an accurate diagnosis in the vast majority of cases. An accurate diagnosis may not be rendered if the specimen is too small or fragmented.

In the above setting, suprabasal acantholysis is diagnostic of PV. Direct immunofluorescence supports the diagnosis by showing IgG and sometimes C3 surrounding epithelial cells.

The differentiation between erosive LP and MP may sometimes not be straightforward. As vesicles are extremely rare in the oral mucosa, in both disorders the exact cause of the erosion may not be apparent in the eroded part of the specimen. The lateral margin, however, may provide some clues. A dense, band-like lymphocytic infiltrate that often contains plasma cells and that may obscure the epithelial basal layer, strongly supports the diagnosis of LP even in the absence of dyskeratosis and basal vacuolization. A partial or complete subepithelial cleft favors MP. The infiltrate in MP is variable and may include lymphocytes, plasma cells, neutrophils, and eosinophils.

In many cases, differentiation between MP and erosive LP is not possible on histological grounds only; hence, the importance of immunofluorescence.

In MP, C3, and IgG are consistently deposited along the basement membrane. Sometimes, IgA is also deposited. Rarely, IgA is the only or the predominant immunoglobulin class rather than IgG. These patients may have IgA MP or mucosal linear IgA disease (also referred to as linear IgA bullous dermatosis). Whether IgA or IgG is the predominant immunoglobulin class, the treatment is the same.

In erosive LP, there is consistent deposition of fibrin along the base of the erosion and the adjacent intact basement membrane. Fibrin deposition is usually intense and markedly thick. Cytoid bodies may also be seen containing IgM.

Conclusions

Patients with a chronic oral erosive eruption are required to have both histological and immunofluorescence evaluation in order to arrive at an accurate diagnosis. It is recommended that biopsies of gingiva and/or palate be performed by an oral surgeon.

Chapter 18
Vulvar Lesions

Figure 18.1 illustrates two patients with two of the disorders discussed in this chapter.

Case A woman presents with persistent vulvar lesion(s). She denies pain.

Clinical Differential Diagnosis and Clinical Clues

The patient denies pain so vulvodynia is excluded. The differential diagnosis varies whether the lesions are papular or patch/plaque.

Papular lesions may be

- condyloma
- Bowenoid Papulosis (BP)
- multiple syringoma, or
- multiple cysts.

Cysts and Syringoma are smooth dermal lesions while condyloma and BP are epidermal.

Although lesions of BP are characterized by a generally smooth surface and reddish brownish color, BP and condyloma cannot be differentiated with absolute certainty based on the clinical examination alone. Syringoma and cysts are both usually multiple and uniformly distributed. Cysts are more likely to be yellowish and round.

Patch lesions may represent

- lichen sclerosis (LS)
- lichen planus (LP) and
- vulvovaginitis,

while plaque lesions may represent

- lichen simplex chronicus (LSC)
- squamous cell carcinoma (SCC) in situ (Bowen disease), and
- extramammary Paget disease (EMPD).

D. F. Mutasim, *Practical Skin Pathology*, DOI 10.1007/978-3-319-14729-1_18

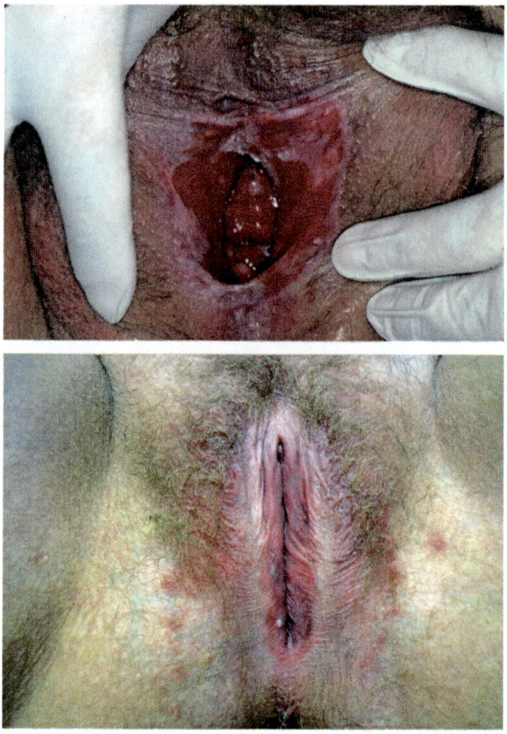

Fig. 18.1 *Upper panel* shows an elderly woman with erosive genital lichen planus presenting with erythema, whitish discoloration, and shallow erosions of the labia minora and vaginal introitus. The patient had oral involvement as well. *Lower panel* shows an elderly woman with well-defined patch of whitish discoloration, atrophy, erythema, telangiectasia, and excoriations characteristic of lichen sclerosis

Lesions of LS are characteristically white with frequent purpura and telangiectasia while lesions of LP are red. Unlike LP involving the penis which presents as papules, LP of the female genitalia presents as red patches. Both disorders involve the labia minora and both may develop erosions. Malignant degeneration is more frequent in lesions of LS. Patients with genital LS may have extragenital lesions, whereas patients with vulvar LP may have oral LP lesions and occasionally lichen planopilaris of the scalp.

Vulvovaginitis may be caused by irritant and/or allergic contact dermatitis as well as Candidal or bacterial infection. Detailed history and complete genital examination, in addition to patch testing and/or cultures, often lead to an accurate diagnosis.

EMPD lesions are generally brightly red and often eroded, and as a result misdiagnosed frequently as Candidiasis. Vulvar SCC in situ may be misdiagnosed as LSC, especially in patients who experience pruritus and admit to scratching which may lead to superimposed lichenification. A high index of suspicion is required for the early diagnosis of EMPD and SCC.

How Helpful Is the Pathology?

very much+++

Normal Histology

The female genital region has significant normal histological variation based on the site being examined. The labia majora are an extension of the adjacent skin and histologically similar to hairy skin, that is, keratinizing squamous epithelium with abundant adnexal structures. The labia minora is non-keratinizing squamous epithelium. The vaginal introitus is lined by mucosal non-keratinizing epithelium. Hence, what is normal for one site may be abnormal for another. When performing a biopsy of female genitalia, an indication of the specific site on the requisition form is essential. The same is true for biopsies of other mucocutaneous junctions such as the penis and lip. (Pathologists often receive a biopsy specimen with the site indicated being simply vulva or lip).

Histological Findings

Papules

Differentiation among the four papular disorders is easy. Keratin *cysts* are similar to epidermoid cysts elsewhere on the body and genital *syringoma* is similar to syringoma elsewhere. *Condyloma* differs from the common wart by having koilocytosis in the mid-layers of the epidermis rather than superficially and having only slight papillomatosis (some genital warts are as papillomatous as verruca vulgaris and are similar clinically to common warts).

Lesions of *BP* may have a similar architecture to condyloma, but in addition have keratinocyte atypia reminiscent of Bowen disease. The degree and extent of atypia, however, varies. Unlike lesions of Bowen disease in which the atypia is severe and uniform among epidermal keratinocytes, the atypia in BP lesions is generally limited to individual scattered keratinocytes throughout hyperplastic, otherwise cytologically unremarkable epidermis. The number of atypical keratinocytes is highly variable and some BP lesions may demonstrate diffuse atypia indistinguishable from Bowen disease. In these cases, clinical correlation is essential. While most patients with BP have multiple lesions, most patients with genital Bowen disease have one lesion only.

Koilocytosis may also be seen in BP, contributing to the possible misdiagnosis of a lesion of BP that demonstrates only minimal keratinocyte atypia as condyloma. If clinical suspicion for BP is high, the dermatologist may obtain further lesions for histological evaluation or request the pathologist to reevaluate sections. It is important to note that some lesions of BP may progress into Bowen disease, especially in the immunocompromised host, such as patients with AIDS.

Patches and Plaques

Lesions of *LS* have easily recognizable and characteristic histological findings. An edematous and progressively hyalinized papillary dermis is sandwiched in between an atrophic overlying epidermis and a band-like lymphocytic infiltrate at the junction between the papillary and superficial particular dermis. Very early lesions, however, may not reveal appreciable epidermal atrophy or papillary dermal changes, making the lymphocytic infiltrate appear band-like immediately beneath the epidermis leading to strong suspicion for LP or less frequently mycosis fungoides. Histological differentiation between LS and LP may be enhanced by identifying an intact basal layer and thin epithelium in LS and indistinct or squamatized basal layer and thick epithelium in LP.

Unlike *LP* papular lesions of the skin and of male genitalia, which almost invariably reveal the well-known characteristic histological findings (compact orthokeratosis, thick granular layer, dyskeratosis, saw-toothing of the tips of the rete, and a dense diffuse band-like lymphocytic infiltrate with several melanophages that hugs and blurs the epidermal basal layer), vulvar LP lesions often lack compact orthokeratosis or a thick granular layer, and the dense lymphocytic infiltrate, although band–like, does not hug and obliterate the epithelial basal layer to the same degree.

Mucosal *pemphigoid* rarely involves the vulvar epithelium without involving other mucous membranes. In difficult or complex cases with no specific diagnosis, pemphigoid should be suspected and immunofluorescence performed, especially if there is evidence of scarring. Erosive vulvar lesions may also be secondary to chronic *HSV* or *CMV* infection.

This is especially true in older and immunosuppressed patients. The characteristic cytopathic changes of acute HSV infection may be absent in chronic HSV infection. Instead, epithelial or epidermal hyperplasia may arise and be severe enough to lead to the wrong diagnosis of an epithelial or epidermal neoplasm. Similarly, chronic erosive CMV infection may be missed histologically unless the diagnosis was suspected and the findings are looked for in multiple sections. (For a discussion of the differential diagnosis of vulvar erosive lesions, the reader is referred to Chap. 17 on oral erosions).

Histological differentiation between *LSC*, *SCC* in situ, and *EMPD* is rather easy. Genital LSC is similar to cutaneous LSC histologically, that is, hyperkeratosis and acanthosis without atypical keratinocytes. Vulvar SCC in situ is similar histologically to cutaneous SCC in situ (epithelial hyperplasia with full-thickness cytological atypia). EMPD reveals single and clustered large round cells with abundant pale cytoplasm throughout the whole thickness of the epithelium. These cells may be identified by regular microscopy easily, and may be confirmed by immunohistochemical markers.

Conclusions

When a woman presents with a complaint related to the genital region, determination is made whether the complaint is:

- Presence of lesions
- Pruritus without lesions (pruritus vulvae-generally idiopathic), or
- Pain or dysesthesia (vulvodynia-often associated with mood disorder)

Common vulvar disorders are often easily identifiable and treatable. Uncommon or persistent lesions in spite of treatment require histological evaluation. Informing the pathologist of the exact site of the biopsy is important.

Chapter 19
Penile Lesions

Figure 19.1 illustrates two patients with two of the disorders discussed in this chapter.

Case A man presents with genital lesions of several weeks to several months duration. Examination reveals papules and/or plaques.

History Elements in the history that are essential to obtain include:

- Age of the patient
- Duration of the lesion(s)
- Symptoms
- Is the patient circumcised?
- Papules versus patch/plaque
- Location of the lesion (glans, prepuce, or skin of the shaft)
- Response to previous treatment
- History of similar lesions or symptoms in members of the household or sexual partners

Clinical Findings Physical findings that may be helpful include:

- Related findings in nongenital skin (such as lesions of psoriasis, scabies, lichen planus (LP), lichen sclerosis (LS), and lichen nitidus (LN))
- Related lesions in adjacent skin such as the scrotum (condyloma, bowenoid papulosis (BP), molluscum, and extramammary Paget disease (EMPD))

Penile lesions of *LP* are more frequently annular and lesions of psoriasis appear less scaly. Patients with genital lesions of scabies almost invariably have lesions elsewhere, and the vast majority of patients with genital psoriasis have psoriasis elsewhere. Genital lesions of *molluscum* are similar to nongenital lesions, but may frequently be pinpoint making differentiation from lichen nitidus and condyloma difficult. Differentiation between *condyloma* and *bowenoid papulosis* (*BP*) is not always possible. Features that raise suspicion for the diagnosis of BP (smooth surface and reddish brown color) are not consistent; hence, requiring a high index of suspicion. Another cause of scaly papular lesions of the penis is *porokeratosis*

D. F. Mutasim, *Practical Skin Pathology*, DOI 10.1007/978-3-319-14729-1_19

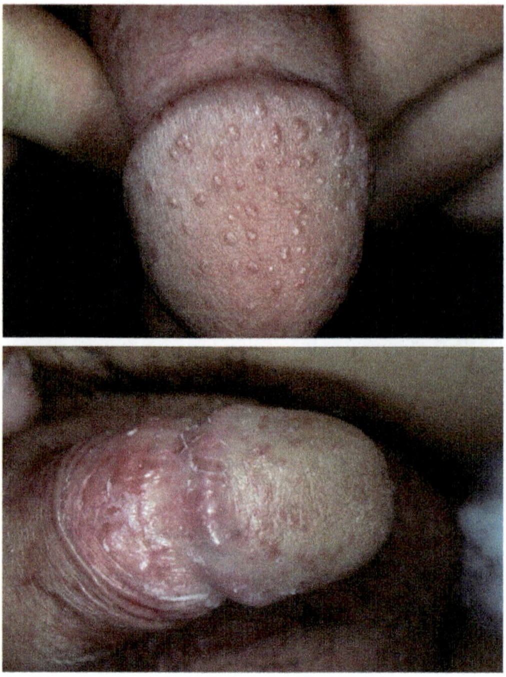

Fig. 19.1 *Upper panel* illustrates penile papules in a young man with severe generalized lichen planus. *Lower panel* illustrates candida balanitis in an older uncircumcised man

pterytropica, a unique type of porokeratosis that involves the anogenital region. Close inspection reveals the characteristic thin keratotic rim at the border. Lesions are sometimes misdiagnosed as psoriasis or condyloma. A biopsy specimen is required to confirm the diagnosis.

A red patch/plaque over the glans penis (which may extend to the prepuce in uncircumcised men) may be inflammatory, infectious, or neoplastic.

Examples of *inflammatory balanitis* include seborrheic balanitis, plasma cell balanitis, and contact balanitis.

Patients with *seborrheic balanitis* often have seborrheic dermatitis elsewhere. History is helpful in confirming the diagnosis of *contact balanitis*. Open patch tests may confirm the diagnosis. A biopsy specimen is often required to confirm the diagnosis of plasma cell balanitis. Some authors argue that *plasma cell balanitis* is not a primary diagnosis but a histological finding in more than one type of balanitis. Others believe that the name describes a specific disorder manifesting as a chronic persistent patch of unknown etiology.

Candidal balanitis, like seborrheic balanitis, is much more common in uncircumcised men. Patients with severe diabetes and immunosuppressed patients are more predisposed for candidal balanitis. The bright red appearance of candidal infection elsewhere is also seen in candidal balanitis. Satellite lesions may be seen as well. Sexual partners of men with candidal balanitis may have candidal vulvovaginitis.

Neoplastic disorders of the glans penis include *SCC* in situ and *EMPD*, and much less frequently other cancers. Both disorders present with a persistent, slowly progressive red patch. Many cases of genital SCC in situ are secondary to HPV infection; hence, other HPV lesions may be present in the immediate vicinity. This is particularly true in immunosuppressed individuals especially the HIV infected who may have several manifestations of HPV infection, including condyloma, BP, and SCC in situ (Bowen disease). In these patients, differentiating a plaque of BP from SCC in situ is not always possible. Immunosuppression is likely to increase the chance of malignant degeneration in lesions of BP.

Both, SCC in situ and EMPD, may occur elsewhere in the anogenital region including the scrotum, groin, and perianal skin.

How Helpful Is the Pathology?

Very much+++

Histological Findings

Most cases of penile papular lesions are diagnosed clinically. If indicated, a biopsy specimen often yields diagnostic results (scabies, LP, LN, psoriasis, condyloma, BP, porokeratosis, and molluscum).

Similarly, most cases of inflammatory and infectious balanitis are diagnosed clinically. Histological examination is less rewarding. The presence of abundant Candidal organisms strongly supports the diagnosis of Candidiasis (a few spores are not sufficient). The presence of a diffuse infiltrate of plasma cells, in the absence of findings characteristic of other disorders, is interpreted as plasma cell balanitis. Contact and seborrheic balanitis are suspected when there is an absence of characteristic findings of other disorders.

Lesions suspected of being neoplastic require histological evaluation, which easily differentiates between SCC in situ and EMPD. When in doubt, immunohistochemical study is helpful.

Other Penile Disorders

The above discussion addressed genital lesions that are persistent and nonulcerative.

Lesions of few days duration that may be vesiculobullous or erosive include HSV infection and fixed drug eruption, which are easily recognizable. Chronic erosive lesions may be caused by chronic HSV infection, chronic CMV infection, and autoimmune bullous disorders such as pemphigus and pemphigoid as well as LP and lichen sclerosis. Cultures and/or immunofluorescence may be needed to confirm the diagnosis.

Conclusions

An accurate diagnosis of penile lesions requires complete skin examination, and occasionally histopathology. The stigma, anxiety, and morbidity that are often associated with genital disorders require that one makes every effort to arrive at a specific diagnosis.

Chapter 20
Diffuse Leg Induration

Figure 20.1 illustrates two patients with two of the disorders discussed in this chapter.

Case A patient presents with diffuse induration of one or both lower legs.
Clinical differential diagnosis includes

- lipodermatosclerosis LDS
- morphea
- necrobiosis lipoidica
- pretibial myxedema, and
- panniculitis..

Clinical Clues

Nodular lesions of *panniculitis* may become confluent, thus giving the impression of diffuse induration; yet it is most likely that one would identify one or few discrete subcutaneous nodules in the vicinity of a large lesion. Pretibial myxedema, panniculitis, and NL are rather easy to diagnose clinically

NL most often presents as a well-defined plaque that is indurated with characteristic color and rarely presents with diffuse induration. It is the only disorder among the six that may spontaneously ulcerate.

Pretibial myxedema is almost always associated with a known thyroid disorder or that may be easily identified by testing at the time of presentation. Unlike the characteristic colors of panniculitis and NL, the skin overlying lesions of pretibial myxedema tends to be normal in color. Unlike lesions in other disorders of this group, lesions of pretibial myxedema tend to be soft or doughy and may show a peau d'orange surface, hypertrichosis, and hyperhidrosis. Massive deposition of mucin focally may result in nodular infiltration within the plaques.

The remaining three disorders in this group are more difficult to distinguish, both, clinically and histologically compared to the above three.

D. F. Mutasim, *Practical Skin Pathology*, DOI 10.1007/978-3-319-14729-1_20

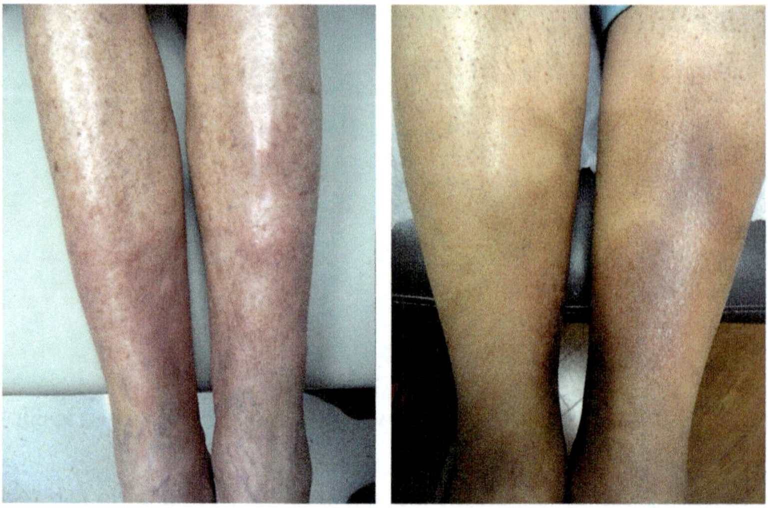

Fig. 20.1 *Upper panel* illustrates an elderly woman with lipodermatosclerosis. Note the brownish discoloration of the indurated skin over the distal lower legs. *Lower panel* illustrates a patient with autoimmune thyroiditis and severe bilateral pretibial myxedema. Note the nodular appearance in addition to the diffuse induration

The most common cause of leg induration today is *LDS*. It is by far more common than morphea and fasciitis. Its incidence has increased rapidly over the last few decades, and likely is secondary to the obesity epidemic. Although LDS may be bilateral, it frequently starts in one leg only for months to years before the other leg becomes involved. Many patients give history of chronic leg edema prior to the onset of manifestations of LDS. Acute LDS is often painful and tender. Severe chronic LDS often acquires an inverted champagne bottle appearance. The diagnosis is generally a clinical one and may be confirmed by histopathology. In most cases, a biopsy is not needed unless there is reason to suspect morphea or fasciitis.

Morphea may be limited to one or occasionally two legs. The most common type of morphea involving the legs is the linear type. The violaceous hue that is characteristic of early-phase plaque morphea is often missing in this form. Unlike LDS, linear morphea of the leg frequently extends to the ankle, foot, and rarely the toes, and is often of the pansclerotic type in which sclerosis is not limited to the reticular dermis, but may involve the fat and extend to the fascia.

Finally, *fasciitis* causes diffuse induration and sclerosis of the legs that the border of involvement may not be easily discernible. The skin surface often becomes irregular.

Three other disorders may result in leg induration, but the lesions are rarely limited to the legs. These are *eosinophilic fasciitis* (which may start on the legs), *scleromyxedema*, and *nephrogenic systemic fibrosis* (*NSF*).

How Helpful Is the Pathology?

Moderately ++

Histological Findings

Histological diagnosis of this group of disorders requires an adequately deep specimen best obtained by the incisional technique.

With rare exception, panniculitis, NL, and pretibial myxedema have characteristic histopathology that is easily differentiated from the other disorders in this group. Rarely, NL may be difficult to differentiate from sarcoidosis or granuloma annulare.

In contradistinction, lesions of LDS, morphea, and fasciitis (especially the latter two) are not as easily distinguishable from each other.

Although *morphea* is primarily a disorder of the reticular dermis and *fasciitis* a disorder of the subcutaneous fascia, the two disorders are not always easily differentiated. This is because the sclerosis of morphea may extend into the subcutaneous fat and superficial fascia (referred to as subcutaneous morphea, morphea profunda, and pansclerotic morphea), and the pathology of fasciitis may extend into the overlying fat and reticular dermis (some refer to this latter presentation as fasciitis with overlying morphea). When dealing with deep induration of the leg, differentiation between fasciitis and deep morphea may be academic.

A 6-mm punch biopsy specimen that contains fat is often adequate to visualize the nonspecific but characteristic findings of LDS. There is variable but generally mild to moderate fibrosis of the deep reticular dermis and fibrous septa of the fat, a minimal or absent infiltrate, and fat degeneration usually resulting in the so-called lipomembranous changes. Although lipomembranous changes are presumed characteristics of LDS, they may be seen in other types of panniculitis.

Conclusions

In the diagnosis of a patient presented with leg induration, a deep elliptical incisional biopsy is required if fasciitis and/or morphea are in the differential diagnosis. Even with an adequate biopsy, differentiation between the two disorders is not always possible. The four other disorders in this group are easy to diagnose.

Chapter 21
Subcutaneous Leg Nodules

Figure 21.1 illustrates two patients with two of the disorders discussed in this chapter.

Case A patient presents with many months history of multiple subcutaneous leg nodules that may wax and wane.

Clinical Differential Diagnosis includes

- panniculitis,
- subcutaneous T-cell lymphoma, and
- infection.

The initial phase of lipodermatosclerosis (LDS) and pretibial myxedema may be nodular.

Clinical Clues The various types of *panniculitis* vary in their preference for sites of involvement (anterior versus posterior legs, overlying joints), whether they involute rapidly or persist for several weeks to a few months, whether they ulcerate or not, and history of apparent precipitating factors or associated systemic disorders. Most types of panniculitis have surface erythema. Occasionally, lesions may become confluent into large plaques.

Dermatology practitioners are generally familiar with the clinical diagnosis of panniculitis. The specific type, however, is not always clinically apparent. When the presentation of subcutaneous leg nodules is acute, strongly favoring the anterior legs, and associated with recent history of infection, pregnancy, or drug use, the diagnosis of erythema nodosum is generally made easily, and a biopsy may not be necessary unless the course of lesions is atypical. All other types of panniculitis require histological confirmation of an adequate biopsy specimen that contains abundant fat.

Panniculitis is traditionally divided into disorders in which the infiltrate primarily involves the lobules of fat and those in which the infiltrate favors the subcutaneous fibrous septae. The prototype of septal panniculitis is erythema nodosum and the prototype of lobular panniculitis is erythema induratum, also referred to by

D. F. Mutasim, *Practical Skin Pathology*, DOI 10.1007/978-3-319-14729-1_21

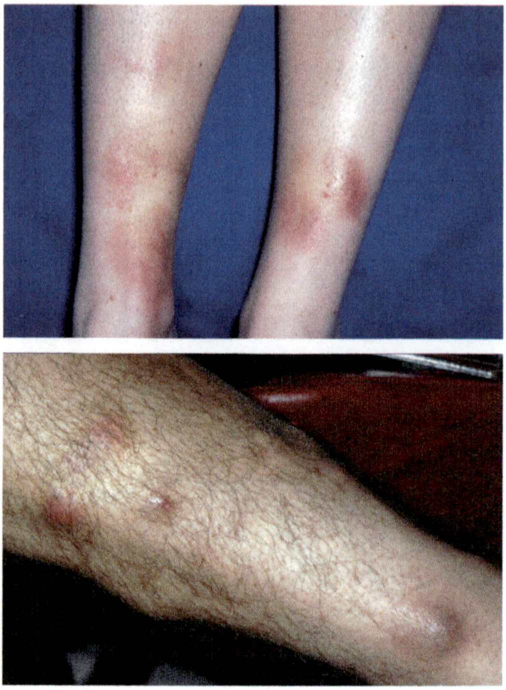

Fig. 21.1 *Upper panel* demonstrates a pregnant woman with classic lesions of erythema nodosum. *Lower panel* demonstrates an elderly man with metastatic colon cancer to the liver resulting in obstruction of the pancreatic duct and secondary pancreatitis and pancreatic panniculitis

some as nodular vasculitis. The latter favors the posterior legs and lesions tend to liquefy and ulcerate. At present, most cases of erythema induratum are idiopathic. Tuberculosis was a common cause when the disorder was initially described several decades ago.

The remaining types of panniculitis are generally rare. Pancreatic panniculitis is usually easily suspected and confirmed. It occurs in patients who generally have known pancreatic disorders or who may have signs and symptoms that point to a pancreatic disorder. Lesions of pancreatic panniculitis often favor the joints. Alpha-1 anti-trypsin deficiency panniculitis is extremely rare, as is eosinophilic panniculitis. Lupus panniculitis is rarely limited to the legs. Most often, it involves the proximal arms and adjacent skin of the shoulders and back, and is almost always followed by a deep indentation at the site of lesions due to atrophy and fibrosis of the subcutaneous fat, which results in "pulling the skin inwards."

When Should an Infection Be Suspected?

Rarely, *bacterial*, *atypical mycobacterial*, and systemic *fungal* infection may present with deep dermal and subcutaneous nodules that may be mistaken clinically for inflammatory panniculitis. Patients are usually immunocompromised such as by HIV infection, immunosuppressive drugs, or chemotherapy.

When Should Subcutaneous T-cell Lymphoma Be Suspected?

Both, T- and B-cell lymphoma have a tendency to involve the leg. A patient with lymphoma of the leg may have diffuse, large B-cell lymphoma (leg type) or subcutaneous T-cell lymphoma. Diffuse, large B-cell lymphoma (leg type) presents as violaceous nodules. In advanced cases, lesions may appear deep and indurated, mimicking other leg disorders.

Subcutaneous T-cell lymphoma, also referred to as subcutaneous panniculitis-like T-cell lymphoma and alpha–beta subcutaneous T-cell lymphoma (referring to the molecular composition of the T-cell receptor) is usually indolent, but may sometimes have an aggressive course.

This is in contrast to T-cell lymphoma that may involve the subcutaneous fat as well as the overlying dermis and epidermis and that carries the T-cell receptor gamma–delta subtype. This disorder used to be referred to as subcutaneous T-cell lymphoma gamma–delta type, but is better referred to as gamma–delta T-cell lymphoma (in order to emphasize the pan-cutaneous nature of the involvement and the fact that the clinical lesions are not subcutaneous nodules, but instead infiltrated and eroded plaques and tumors). Gamma–delta T-cell lymphoma carries a poor prognosis, often associated with the hemophagocytic syndrome and death.

Clues to suspecting subcutaneous T-cell lymphoma include persistence of lesions for several months, lack of spontaneous involution, and continued progression of lesions in a patient with subcutaneous leg nodules without identifiable cause.

How Helpful Is the Pathology?

Very helpful+++

Histological Clues

Histologically, classic erythema nodosum and classic erythema induratum are easily identifiable. *Erythema nodosum* is characterized by septal widening and an infiltrate of multinucleated cells, neutrophils, and lymphocytes, and minimal involvement of the periphery of fat lobules. Difficulties in the diagnosis of erythema nodosum may occur in small specimens, superficial specimens that include only little fat or in involuting lesions.

Erythema induratum is characterized by medium-sized vessel vasculitis, granulomatous inflammation, and necrosis. Difficulty in making the diagnosis of erythema induratum may result from an inadequate biopsy specimen but also may be due to the variability in the presence and degree of each of the three characteristic findings of the disorder. In some cases, vasculitis of medium-sized vessels is the most prominent finding, leading some to use the term *nodular vasculitis* as synonymous with erythema induratum.

Some have advocated that lesions with prominent necrosis and granulomatous inflammation are more likely to be caused by tuberculosis and should be referred to as erythema induratum of Bazin in honor of Dr. Bazin, who first described the condition in association with and as a distant reaction to tuberculosis, a tuberculid. In this latter analysis, the term nodular vasculitis was suggested to be reserved for those lesions that were not associated with tuberculosis. For practical purposes, patients whose biopsies are interpreted as erythema induratum or nodular vasculitis need to be evaluated for tuberculosis by the PPD test and x-ray of the chest as well as other systemic causes.

The characteristic histological findings of *Lupus panniculitis* vary with the age of the lesion. Early lesions are characterized by a lobular lymphocytic infiltrate that may contain plasma cells and/or lymphoid follicles, and deposition of mucin in the deep dermis and subcutaneous fat. As lesions age, the intensity of the infiltrate decreases and the mucin deposition is gradually replaced by collagen deposition leading finally to the histological findings of the so-called sclerosing panniculitis (a histological rather than a clinical term), which causes the characteristic indentation in involuting lesions of Lupus panniculitis.

Another inflammatory disorder that causes subcutaneous nodules over the legs is *cutaneous polyarteritis nodosa* (*PAN*). A clue to the clinical diagnosis is the frequent association with livedo reticularis. The initial phase of blood vessel wall inflammation is neutrophilic while later phases become predominantly histiocytic.

Panniculitis secondary to *alpha-1 anti-trypsin deficiency* reveals a neutrophilic infiltrate in the superficial fat and fat–dermal junction; hence, requiring a high index of suspicion. A diffuse infiltrate of neutrophils in the fat in the absence of superficial dermal neutrophilic infiltrate likely represents *subcutaneous Sweet syndrome*. Patients with subcutaneous Sweet syndrome have lesions that look similar to those of classic Sweet syndrome. Liquifactive fat necrosis with ghost cells is characteristic of *Pancreatic panniculitis*, and is easily identifiable. *Eosinophilic panniculitis* is a rare disorder in which the fat is infiltrated diffusely by eosinophils, making the diagnosis easy. Caution should be exercised in biopsies of insect bite reaction in which the dermal eosinophilic infiltrate extends into the subcutaneous fat. The findings in LDS are discussed in Chap. 20 on "leg induration."

Infection and foreign body reaction are suspected histologically in the presence of overlying dermal involvement, necrosis, and the presence of, both, suppurative and granulomatous inflammation. Special stains may be helpful especially in fungal infections. Tissue cultures are required.

Subcutaneous T-cell lymphoma (alpha-beta type) presents histologically with a lymphocytic infiltrate in the fat without vasculitis, granulomatous inflammation, or necrosis. Very mild fat degeneration may be present. The intensity of the lobular lymphocytic infiltrate varies from mild to severe. In some cases, a rim of lymphocytes surrounding individual fat cells is seen and easily alerts the pathologist about the diagnosis. In many cases, however, the finding is missing and clues to suspecting the diagnosis include:

- An exclusively or predominantly lymphocytic infiltrate that is generally monomorphic
- The infiltrate lacking significant atypia so that its malignant nature may be missed, and
- Absence of characteristics of inflammatory panniculitis

In suspected cases, immunohistochemical studies may be helpful and submitting tissue for TCR monoclonality is usually positive and confirms the diagnosis.

What Is the Relationship Between Lupus Panniculitis and Subcutaneous T-cell Lymphoma?

In the past few years, some have proposed that Lupus panniculitis and subcutaneous T-cell lymphoma are the two ends of a spectrum. Reasons presented for the argument include the observations that:

- Both disorders result from infiltration of the fat by T-cells
- Some cases of Lupus panniculitis reveal monoclonality of the T-cells
- Some cases that were initially diagnosed histologically as Lupus panniculitis were ultimately confirmed to be subcutaneous T-cell lymphoma

Based on these observations, some have proposed that Lupus panniculitis may be a precursor for subcutaneous T-cell lymphoma.

In the author's clinical and pathology experience, no patient diagnosed initially with Lupus panniculitis has ever progressed to subcutaneous T-cell lymphoma over a period of up to 25 years. While subcutaneous T-cell lymphoma strongly favors the lower extremities, Lupus panniculitis is either generalized or more frequently limited to the shoulder girdle area.

So, should cases diagnosed histologically as lupus panniculitis be further investigated for TCR clonality; and, should patients be observed closely and biopsied frequently?

I believe that most pathologists would answer in the negative. Cases with classic clinical and histological findings of Lupus panniculitis do not require evaluation for lymphoma but instead for SLE as some patients with Lupus panniculitis may have systemic involvement.

Instead, a histological diagnosis of "nonspecific panniculitis" or "lymphocytic panniculitis" requires further evaluation for the possibility of subcutaneous T-cell lymphoma or lupus panniculitis by obtaining an adequate-sized biopsy specimen of a "mature" lesion, neither too early nor too old.

How About the Coexistence of Lesions of Lupus Panniculitis and DLE Within the Same Site?

Some references report that the findings of overlying discoid lupus erythematosus (DLE) are present in approximately half of the lesions of Lupus panniculitis. This is greatly exaggerated. Almost all patients who present with clinically classic Lupus panniculitis do not have the characteristic changes of overlying DLE clinically or histologically. In contrast, in a number of biopsy specimens of patients with active DLE, the dermal lymphocytic infiltrate extends into the fat. In these cases, fat involvement is merely an extension of the deep dermal infiltrate into the adjacent superficial fat; lymphoid follicles and fat hyalinization are not seen. These cases are best viewed as DLE with additional fat involvement instead of lupus panniculitis with overlying DLE. In the author's experience, these patients usually have the clinical appearance of DLE, but with the additional finding that lesions are more boggy or indurated than classic DLE lesions.

Conclusions

In the workup of patients with leg nodules, any combination of the following may be needed to arrive at an accurate diagnosis:

- Adequate preferably incisional biopsy containing abundant fat
- Special stains
- Immunohistochemistry
- Molecular testing for TCR clonality, and
- Evaluation for systemic disorders

A histological diagnosis of "nonspecific panniculitis" or "lymphocytic panniculitis" requires further evaluation.

Chapter 22
Leg Ulcers

Figure 22.1 illustrates two patients with two of the disorders discussed in this chapter.

Case An obese, diabetic 65-year-old presents with a chronic, persistent lower leg ulcer. The patient reports minor trauma at the onset of the ulcer. Patient reports two similar lesions, both following trauma but that healed within a few weeks, two years earlier.

The clinical differential diagnosis includes

- venous ulcer
- diabetic ulcer,
- arterial ulcer,
- ulcerating pyoderma gangrenosum (PG),
- occlusive vasculopathy, and
- traumatic/self-induced ulcer.

The history of recurrence precludes ulcerating carcinoma or infection (both being rare causes of leg ulcers). By far, the most common cause of leg ulcers is venous insufficiency, and attempts to confirm or exclude the diagnosis are essential.

Clinical Clues

Clinical clues for the possible diagnosis include:

- The location of the ulcer
- The morphology of the base
- The morphology of the border
- Severity of pain
- The presence of specific findings of arterial or venous insufficiency in the adjacent skin of the lower leg

D. F. Mutasim, *Practical Skin Pathology*, DOI 10.1007/978-3-319-14729-1_22

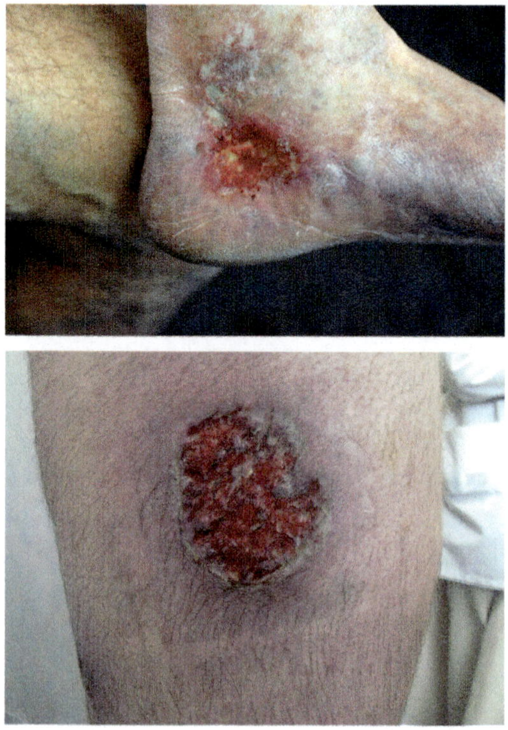

Fig. 22.1 *Upper panel* shows an elderly man with chronic painful ulcer over the lower medial ankle with histological findings of hyalinizing vasculitis. Note the surrounding atrophy, whitish discoloration, and telangiectasia characteristic of atrophie blanche. *Lower panel* shows the lower leg of a young man with ulcerative colitis and pyoderma gangrenosum

Location of the Ulcer

Ulcers secondary to venous insufficiency strongly favor the inner or medial ankle overlying the site of the incompetent vein. Arterial ulcers in contrast favor the outer or lateral ankle. Diabetic ulcers favor pressure points of the feet, and are characteristically surrounded by callus tissue due to a walking deformity, secondary to diabetic neuropathy. Ulcers secondary to occlusive vasculopathy, such as anti-phospholipid antibodies or secondary to hyalinizing vasculitis, have no striking preference between the medial or lateral ankle. Also, ulcers secondary to PG do not have site preference over the leg.

Morphology of the Base

Arterial and diabetic ulcers tend to be much deeper and have a punched-out appearance than ulcers due to venous insufficiency and occlusive vasculopathy. All ulcers may have a moist or dry base and a variable degree of granulation tissue based on the duration of the ulcer and its management so far.

Morphology of the Border

The border of arterial and diabetic ulcers tends to be punched out, while that of a venous ulcer tends to be ragged. The ulcers secondary to PG have a characteristic violaceous edematous border with a variable degree of undermining. PG ulcers are more likely to heal with cribriform scarring.

The ulcers of hyalinizing vasculitis are often surrounded by purpura, just as ulcers secondary to vasculitis. Although vasculitis may result in leg ulcers, vasculitis presenting as a solitary ulcerating lesion is extremely rare. I have seen two such cases both secondary to rheumatoid vasculitis, but the presentation was that of a purpuric plaque with ulceration.

A geographic or figurate shape, especially in the absence of significant or commensurate pain, should raise suspicion for a self-induced ulcer.

Severity of Pain

In general, arterial ulcers are extremely painful and venous ulcers only slightly. Pain secondary to PG is variable, ranging from mild to excruciating. Ulcers secondary to hyalinizing vasculitis are generally extremely painful; few patients report only mild pain. Self-induced ulcers should be considered in the absence of pain or if the patient's affect is incommensurate with the apparent severity of the ulcer.

Skin Findings Adjacent to the Ulcer

Skin changes of venous insufficiency are well known, and include leg edema that is worse as the day goes by, superficial varicosities, petechiae, and discoloration secondary to iron deposition. Any number of these findings may be present, but none is absolutely necessary or sufficient to make the diagnosis of venous ulcer. Venous hypertension may be present in the absence of these clinical findings.

The skin changes of the legs in patients with arterial insufficiency are also well known and include loss of hair, dryness, and peripheral pallor and/or cyanosis.

The skin immediately surrounding ulcers secondary to PG may have a violaceous hue, while the skin surrounding lesions of chronic occlusive vasculopathy (especially hyalinizing vasculitis) often reveals porcelain white scarring with surrounding telangiectasias and faint erythema, so-called "*atrophie blanche.*"

Active or healing excoriations adjacent to an ulcer raise suspicion for traumatic cause.

How Helpful Is the Pathology?

Moderately +/++

Histological Clues

In early or active lesions of *PG*, a biopsy specimen from the border of the lesion is likely to reveal the characteristic findings of a dense and diffuse neutrophilic infiltrate spanning the whole dermis and associated with necrosis and secondary ulceration. Blood vessel walls may be trapped in the infiltrate thus appearing vasculitic. In late lesions of PG in which the border does not retain the characteristic clinical appearance, the histological findings are likely to be nonspecific and often cannot be differentiated from ulcers secondary to venous insufficiency. A neutrophilic infiltrate at the base of an ulcer may be seen in a chronic ulcer secondary to multiple causes, and does not imply PG or secondary bacterial infection. Neutrophils are an integral part of the initial inflammatory phase of wound healing.

The presence of histological findings of *venous insufficiency* (that is, groups of proliferating superficial venules and capillaries) is not diagnostic of venous ulcer. Histological evidence of venous insufficiency may be present in lower leg biopsies after the third decade of life without necessarily being associated with clinically significant venous disease. In venous ulcers, progressive occlusion of the superficial vessel walls by fibrinous material may be easily evident histologically, and helps support the clinical diagnosis. In order to confirm the diagnosis of venous ulcer, findings of other causes of leg ulcers should be absent. Evidence of venous hypertension should be sought after by venous ultrasound (that is Doppler studies).

In general, *arterial ulcers* are deeper than venous ulcers. Their location and associated severe pain, especially in a patient with evidence of peripheral atherosclerosis are often sufficient and a biopsy is generally avoided. There are no diagnostic histological characteristics of arterial ulcers. The diagnosis is confirmed by arterial studies, both, by ultrasound and radiography.

Conclusions

In many patients with a leg ulcer, an accurate diagnosis may be made by obtaining a detailed history, physical examination, and evaluation for arterial and/or venous insufficiency.

Since the treatment of each of the causes of leg ulcers is unique, a search for the diagnosis of PG is justified. The diagnosis of PG may be made clinically in the early or acute stage of the lesion especially in the presence of an associated systemic illness including inflammatory bowel disease in up to 50% of the patients, and excluding the other causes of leg ulcers.

Venous ulcers are much more common than arterial ulcers in dermatology practice. Since the treatment of the two is quite different, arterial evaluation may be recommended in patients who appear to have venous ulcers but in whom the severity of the pain is high, or in whom, compression and other modalities of treating a venous ulcer have not been sufficient.

Although the changes of *atrophie blanche* are assumed to be characteristic of hyalinizing vasculitis, similar findings may be seen in the healing phases of venous ulcers. Hence, *atrophie blanche* should not be equated with hyalinizing vasculitis, but instead as a morphological clinical finding in the healing of some leg ulcers.

Chapter 23
Follicular Papules and Pustules—Trunk

Figure 23.1 illustrates two patients with two of the disorders discussed in this chapter.

Case A patient presents with a chronic eruption of papules and pustules favoring the trunk especially the back with follicular appearance.

Clinical differential diagnosis includes

- acne,
- bacterial folliculitis,
- Pityrosporum folliculitis, and
- eosinophilic folliculitis.

Clinical Clues

Papulo-pustular *acne* limited to the back or upper trunk with no involvement of the face is rare. In the presence of comedones, the diagnosis of acne may be easily made. However, comedones may be missing, making the diagnosis of acne somewhat difficult without histological evaluation. This is especially true if the onset of the eruption is delayed beyond the acne age. In such cases, the differential diagnosis would include bacterial and Pityrosporum folliculitis, and eosinophilic folliculitis. Acne is strongly suspected in the presence of nodular/cystic lesions.

Unlike cases of facial *eosinophilic folliculitis*, those with trunk involvement are much more likely to have associated immunosuppression. Lesions tend to be pruritic and pustules may decorate the border of an annular plaque. In HIV-positive individuals, lesions of eosinophilic folliculitis often are difficult to distinguish from the so-called papular eruption of HIV disease. Some authors believe that the two disorders may be related or may coexist based on examining multiple biopsies from the same patient.

D. F. Mutasim, *Practical Skin Pathology*, DOI 10.1007/978-3-319-14729-1_23

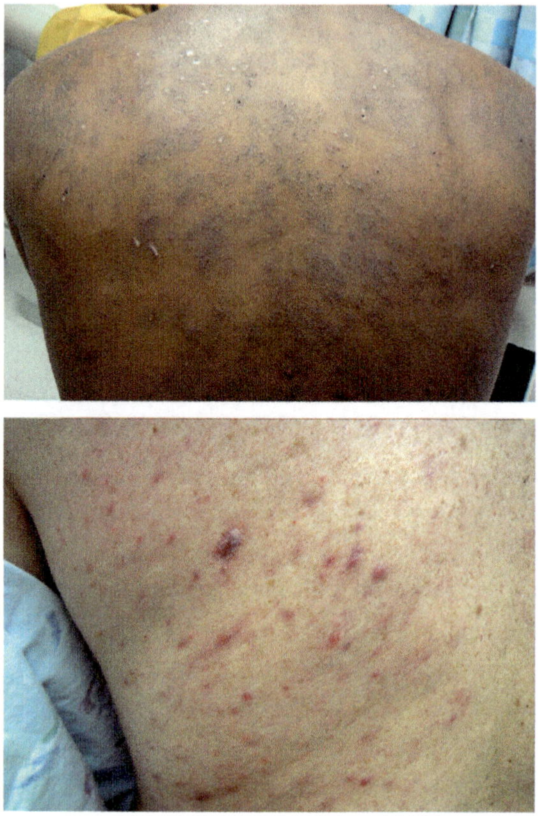

Fig. 23.1 *Upper panel* shows an HIV-positive man with hyperpigmented macules and several scattered pustules, many at the borders of the macules. Histological examination confirmed the diagnosis of eosinophilic folliculitis. *Lower panel* shows an obese middle-aged man with numerous purplish papulopustules over the trunk. Biopsy specimen revealed pityrosporum folliculitis

Chronic bacterial folliculitis is often associated with furuncles, and less commonly with carbuncles. Lesions of bacterial folliculitis are often painful or burning. Lesions are generally brightly red papules surmounted by a pustule. Lesions may favor areas predisposed to friction or occlusion such as the buttock and posterior thigh.

Lesions of *Pityrosporum folliculitis*, although caused by the same organism as tinea versicolor, are very rarely associated with the characteristic finely scaling eruption. Like bacterial folliculitis, conditions that contribute to the development of Pityrosporum folliculitis include heat, humidity and increased sweating, and occlusion. Unlike lesions of bacterial folliculitis, which are characteristically striking pustules with red halos, lesions of Pityrosporum folliculitis are much more persistent, acquiring purplish and brownish hues reflecting granulomatous inflammation histologically.

How Helpful Is the Pathology?

Moderately ++

Histological Clues

Papules and pustules of *acne* share with infectious folliculitis histological features of a ruptured hair follicle surrounded by a variably mixed infiltrate of neutrophils, histiocytes, and multinucleated cells. Histological confirmation of the diagnosis of acne requires the finding of comedonal, rounded dilatation of the follicular infundibulum. In the absence of this finding, a diagnosis of acne can only be suspected but not confirmed with certainty.

Bacterial folliculitis usually reveals a dense collection of neutrophils (pustule) in the superficial follicular epithelium (infundibulum), and sometimes the mid- and dccp portions as well.

Pityrosporum folliculitis tends to reveal in addition to neutrophils, histiocytes, and sometimes multinucleated giant cells. Spores are usually seen in the dilated superficial portion of the follicular epithelium. The mere presence of a few spores in a dilated infundibulum in a lesion of folliculitis does not confirm the diagnosis of pityrosporum folliculitis. Pityrosporum spores may be seen in otherwise normal hair follicles and those affected by other types of folliculitis.

Eosinophilic folliculitis is characterized by an infiltrate rich in eosinophils in and around follicular epithelium, adjacent dermis, and sometimes the overlying epidermis. This presumes the presence of a hair follicle in the examined sections, which sometimes may be missed by the biopsy procedure or sectioning; hence, emphasizing the need for two or more biopsies. It has been reported that unlike lesions of eosinophilic folliculitis of the face in which follicular involvement is frequently detected, the infiltrate in eosinophilic folliculitis of the trunk may not involve a hair follicle. Some may not accept the diagnosis of eosinophilic folliculitis in the absence of documented follicular involvement.

The author has seen cases of a papular pustular eruption over the back of HIV-positive men in whom one of the two biopsies reveals follicular involvement and the other does not. Hence, if only one biopsy specimen is obtained and it did not reveal follicular enforcement, the histological diagnosis given may be that of a dermal hypersensitivity reaction or the papular eruption of HIV disease by some and as consistent with eosinophilic folliculitis (without follicular involvement) by others. The two types of lesions produce similar symptoms and respond to similar treatments. Whether patients with HIV infection have one or more eosinophilic disorder resulting in pruritic papules of the trunk may be further elucidated when the cause of both presentations is known.

Conclusions

In the histological evaluation of a patient with papulopustules over the trunk, two or more biopsies are more likely to result in making an accurate diagnosis.

Chapter 24
Palmoplantar Red Hyperkeratosis

Figure 24.1 illustrates two patients with two of the disorders discussed in this chapter.

Case A patient presents with an acquired bilateral reddish scaly or hyperkeratotic eruption of the palms, with or without plantar involvement.

This presentation may overlap with inherited palmoplantar keratodermas (PPK), and be confused with them in the absence of personal and family history. In this section, the inherited keratodermas will not be addressed. *Clinical differential diagnosis* includes

- palmoplantar plaque psoriasis,
- chronic hand dermatitis (usually referring to chronic irritant hand dermatitis),
- a subtype of chronic hand dermatitis referred to as "chronic hyperkeratotic eczema (CHE),"
- palmoplantar discoid lupus erythematosus
- discoid lupus erythematosus (DLE) and
- tinea.

Tinea, psoriasis and CHE may involve the soles of the feet.

Rarely, a patient with the above clinical presentation may be harboring mycosis fungoides (MF) and much more rarely a paraneoplastic disorder (paraneoplastic palmoplantar keratoderma). Patients with pityriasis rubra pilaris (PRP) and papulosquamous-secondary syphilis who have palmoplantar involvement are easily diagnosed on the basis of having other manifestations of PRP and syphilis.

The most common differential diagnosis submitted with a biopsy specimen from the palm or sole is dermatitis, tinea, and psoriasis. If there are coexisting pustules the differential diagnosis is palmoplantar pustular psoriasis and tinea, and less frequently dermatitis with secondary bacterial infection. Clinical Clues

Tinea is strongly suspected if the hand involvement is unilateral, especially in the presence of bilateral plantar involvement (the so-called two-foot, one-hand tinea). Palmoplantar tinea varies in clinical morphology from fine scaling and desquamation (a common presentation in asymptomatic patients) to redness and scaling to pustules

D. F. Mutasim, *Practical Skin Pathology*, DOI 10.1007/978-3-319-14729-1_24

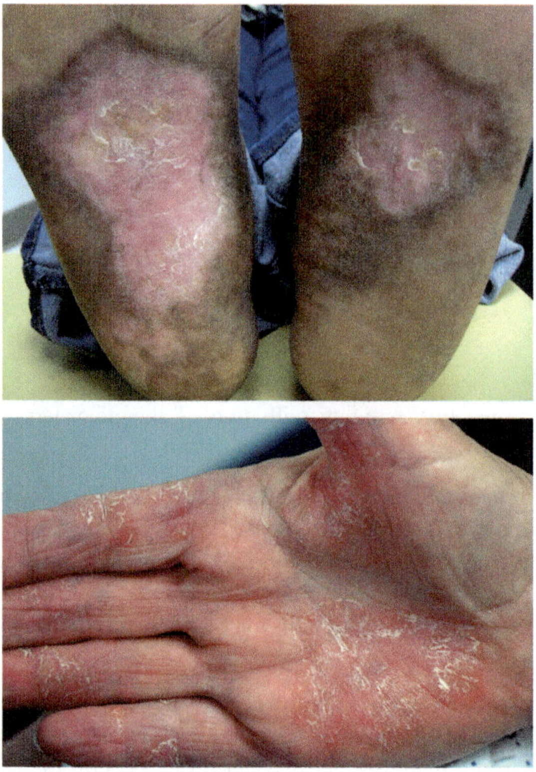

Fig. 24.1 *Upper panel* demonstrates a young African–American woman with palmoplantar discoid lupus erythematosus. Note the loss of pigmentation, erythema, and hyperkeratosis at the center and hyperpigmentation at the periphery. *Lower panel* demonstrates discrete reddish hyperkeratotic plaques limited to the palms in a patient with chronic hyperkeratotic eczema

and bullae. An active inflammatory border may be seen. Some nails, especially toenails, may show evidence of onychomycosis.

Plaque psoriasis of the palms and soles is very close in clinical appearance to that of plaque psoriasis on other parts of the skin surface. Occasionally, patients with palmoplantar plaque psoriasis may have mild lesions on the elbows, knees, or scalp which they may not be aware of. If present, characteristic nail changes are helpful in confirming the diagnosis of psoriasis.

Lesions of DLE often are hypopigmented, atrophic and have an infiltrated border. So-called *chronic hand dermatitis* (either solely or partially due to chronic irritancy) almost universally demonstrates dorsal hand involvement. The diagnosis may be further supported in patients who report previous history of atopic dermatitis or who wash their hands frequently. Fissuring and fingertip involvement is common.

CHE involves the palms more than the soles. Plantar involvement is invariably accompanied by palmar involvement. Lesions are intermediate in morphology between palmar psoriasis and chronic hand dermatitis. The hyperkeratosis is characteristically compact, almost waxy. CHE may be viewed both clinically and histologically as intermediate between chronic hand dermatitis and palmar psoriasis. The exact nosology of CHE, and its possible relation to psoriasis and chronic hand dermatitis is not known.

CHE is often asymptomatic and often associated with repetitive trauma of work or sport activities. The lesions are more hyperkeratotic than chronic hand dermatitis, and often in the form of a few, large plaques rather than diffuse involvement of the palm. The hyperkeratosis tends to be compact. Attempts at scraping the surface for microscopic examination are often unyielding, unlike the case in patients with tinea or psoriasis.

In my experience, a rare patient carried with the diagnosis of palmar CHE has shown evidence of plaque psoriasis elsewhere 10 years or longer after the onset of palmar involvement. Continual search for evidence of psoriasis in patients with CHE may help delineate those patients with "CHE" who are harbingers of psoriasis or those who may be viewed as having undiagnosed psoriasis from the beginning.

The cases in which the clinical diagnosis is not clearly apparent, practitioners often ask for help from the pathologist.

How Helpful Is the Pathology?

At best, moderate++

Common Disorders

Histological findings overlap among the above disorders.

Plaque psoriasis of the palms and soles may not reveal the same characteristic findings seen in plaque psoriasis elsewhere. In other words, histological findings in plaque psoriasis of the palms and soles are generally "imperfect" or "incomplete." Parakeratosis is often focal rather than diffuse; the granular layer not absent throughout; spongiosis and serum in the stratum corneum may be present, and neutrophilic collections are not as discrete as in plaque psoriasis. The diagnosis, however, can be strongly suspected if the findings of the other disorders, for example, fungal organisms or significant spongiosis, are absent.

Tinea is suspected in the presence of neutrophils in the horny layer and the diagnosis is confirmed by special stains.

Chronic hand dermatitis may reveal findings of both irritant dermatitis (superficial epidermal degeneration with or without neutrophils and variable epidermal hyperplasia) and spongiotic dermatitis.

CHE demonstrates hyperkeratosis, usually compact, acanthosis, and generally mild or no spongiosis.

Uncommon Disorders

A rare patient who carries a diagnosis of chronic hand dermatitis will have *MF* upon further evaluation. Lesions of palmoplantar MF may be scaly, hyperkeratotic, or vesiculopustular; hence, the diagnosis may be missed for other common disorders such as hand dermatitis, psoriasis, and tinea. Since the histology mimics the clinical findings, MF may also be missed histologically, especially if there is severe spongiosis.

One of the most concerning but extremely rare causes of palmoplantar red hyperkeratosis is "paraneoplastic palmoplantar keratoderma." The disorder does not have histological characteristics but is suspected clinically when palmoplantar keratoderma is of late onset and has a rapid onset and progression.

Conclusions

In approaching the diagnosis of a patient with palmar or palmoplantar eruption, history and physical examination with reference to signs of disease elsewhere may be sufficient. When a patient does not respond to treatment as expected, a biopsy specimen may be necessary.

Chapter 25
Skin Folds Diffuse Rash

Figure 25.1 illustrates two patients with two of the disorders discussed in this chapter.

Case A patient presents with a chronic rash of the groin with or without involvement of other skin folds.

Clinical differential diagnosis includes

- intertrigo
- candidiasis
- erythrasma
- tinea
- gram-negative infection (especially in toe web maceration)
- psoriasis
- chronic dermatitis
- Hailey–Hailey disease (HHD), and
- granular parakeratosis.

Disorders which present with papules, such as condyloma, molluscum, skin tags, groin acantholytic dermatosis, or nodules, such as hidradenitis, are not considered here.

Clinical Clues

History

It is highly likely to elicit a positive family history in HHD and to a lesser degree in psoriasis. Patients with intertrigo and candidiasis are more likely to be overweight or obese. Patients with tinea and chronic dermatitis are more likely to report pruritus.

D. F. Mutasim, *Practical Skin Pathology*, DOI 10.1007/978-3-319-14729-1_25

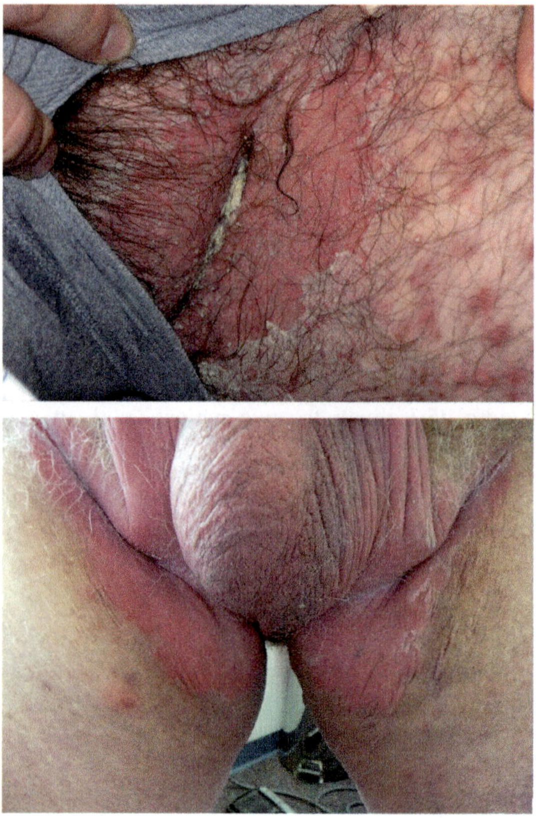

Fig. 25.1 *Upper panel* represents a 20-year-old man with pemphigus vulgaris who was in remission on immunosuppressive therapy and presented with a "flare of his disease." Histological evaluation confirmed the clinical diagnosis of candidiasis. *Lower panel* represents a middle-aged man with flexural psoriasis. Note the well-defined nature of the plaques

Examination

Upon examination, the lesions are:

- More likely to be well defined in psoriasis, tinea, and erythrasma; and ill-defined in intertrigo, candidiasis, and chronic dermatitis
- More likely to be crusted and/or vesicular in HHD and have active (pustular, vesicular, scaly) border in tinea
- Generally brightly red in psoriasis, candidiasis, and HHD, and brown in erythrasma and granular parakeratosis
- Usually raised in HHD, psoriasis, chronic dermatitis, and granular parakeratosis, and more flat in intertrigo, candidiasis, and erythrasma

Patients with psoriasis and HHD are more likely to have involvement of multiple skin folds.

Limitations in Clinical Diagnosis

In spite of the above clues, a clinical diagnosis is not always possible due to several reasons:

1. Two disorders may overlap in the same patient. For example, patients with flexural psoriasis who experience pruritus may develop overlying lichenification. They may also develop secondary candidal or bacterial infection.
2. Partial treatment or the use of OTC preparations, including excessive use of detergents or rubbing alcohol, may also modify the clinical appearance of flexural disorders.
3. Chronic HHD may present with papules and/or plaques with no clinical evidence of vesiculation or crusting, closely mimicking chronic lesions of Darier disease.
4. Candidiasis may not have satellite lesions and may rarely present with multiple discrete annular lesions, with superficial sloughing of the border reminiscent of impetigo.
5. Candidiasis without satellite lesions may be misdiagnosed as simple intertrigo.
6. What appears as possible tinea or simple intertrigo of the toe webs may instead be gram-negative toe web infection or complex infection by multiple organisms.
7. Erythema of the perianal skin, which may be misdiagnosed as intertrigo or candidiasis, may represent streptococcal cellulitis.
8. Having minimal physical findings in the groin of someone complaining of pruritus may be due to partially suppressed tinea (tinea incognito).

How Helpful Is the Pathology?

Moderately helpful++

Histological Clues

The histological findings in HHD and granular parakeratosis are characteristic and easily identifiable.

Full thickness intraepidermal acantholysis in a pattern of "dilapidated brick wall" is diagnostic of *HHD* in the proper clinical setting. Groin acantholytic disorder may be difficult to distinguish but is more likely to reveal dyskeratosis and presents with papules instead. The histological differential diagnosis also includes pemphigus vulgaris and pemphigus vegetans. Patients with pemphigus vulgaris consistently have lesions elsewhere. Lesions of pemphigus vegetans may be limited to the skin folds only. Pemphigus vegetans is more likely to reveal epithelial and follicular epithelial hyperplasia. If in doubt, immunofluorescence may need to be performed.

Granular parakeratosis is characterized by a thick layer of parakeratosis with retention of keratohyalin granules in the parakeratotic corneocytes, and prominent nuclei in the superficial granular cells.

The histological findings of other flexural disorders are generally less characteristic and sometimes non-diagnostic.

Lesions of *flexural psoriasis* may reveal histological findings similar to those of plaque psoriasis elsewhere, especially if not treated and not lichenified. Often, however, the findings are "less perfect" than in plaque psoriasis. Because of the occlusive, moist nature of the lesions, the stratum corneum may be decreased or lost due to maceration. The presence of neutrophils in the stratum corneum of the groin or other flexural skin may not carry the diagnostic significance that it does in plaque psoriasis. Neutrophils may be seen on the surface of lesions of intertrigo, candidiasis, tinea, and dermatitis. The most reliable findings for the diagnosis of flexural psoriasis may be loss of the granular layer and regular epidermal hyperplasia in the absence of evidence for candidiasis or tinea.

Tinea and *candidiasis* may share histological findings, namely, features of subacute or chronic dermatitis with neutrophils in the stratum corneum and/or superficial epidermis. The two disorders are differentiated by special stains that highlight the organisms.

The histological findings in *intertrigo* and *erythrasma* are those of mild dermatitis and are nonspecific. It is extremely rare that a biopsy is obtained to confirm or exclude either diagnosis. Findings in *chronic dermatitis* are similar to those of chronic dermatitis elsewhere, namely, hyperkeratosis, acanthosis, and a lymphocytic infiltrate.

Conclusions

Multiple disorders may involve flexural skin. Genital disorders that may extend to the groin are addressed separately (Chaps. 18 and 19). Differentiating among flexural disorders based on clinical findings alone is possible in the majority of patients. Histological evaluation is helpful in the remaining minority.

Chapter 26
Exfoliative Erythroderma

Figure 26.1 illustrates two patients with two of the disorders discussed in this chapter.

Case A patient presents with rapidly progressive eruption. Examination reveals total skin redness and scaling.

Clinical differential diagnosis includes

- psoriasis
- pityriasis rubra pilaris (PRP)
- atopic dermatitis
- Sezary syndrome (SS)
- drug-induced erythroderma
- crusted scabies, and rarely
- pemphigus foliaceous (PF).

The discussion is limited to acquired primary skin disorders that may present with exfoliative erythroderma. Other disorders that may present with exfoliative erythroderma include some types of ichthyosis. As these are known since early childhood, they are not discussed here. Erythroderma secondary to viral or bacterial exanthem is generally without scaling and patients usually have systemic symptoms, and will not be discussed here. Also, morbilliform drug eruption that may show fine desquamation as the eruption involutes will not be discussed.

Clinical Clues

History

Patients with exfoliative erythroderma secondary to psoriasis, atopic dermatitis, crusted scabies, and pemphigus foliaceous generally have a preceding limited skin disorder for weeks to years before advancing to total skin involvement. On the other hand, exfoliative erythroderma secondary to drug-induced or Sezary syndrome is

D. F. Mutasim, *Practical Skin Pathology*, DOI 10.1007/978-3-319-14729-1_26

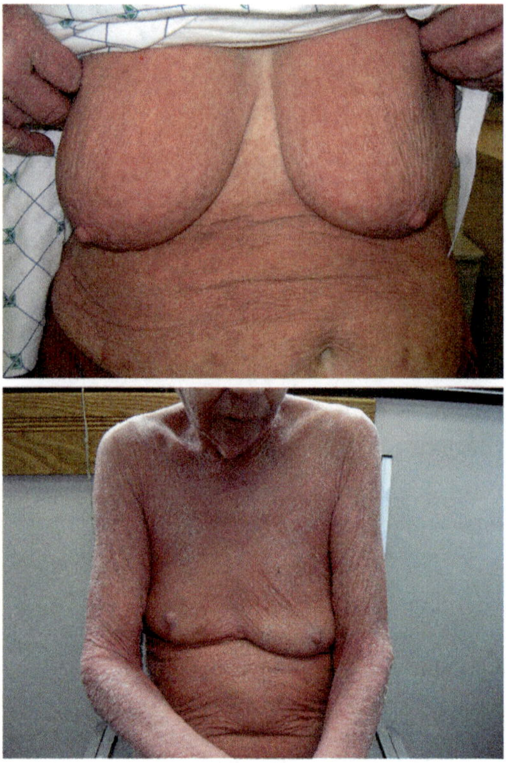

Fig. 26.1 *Upper panel* illustrates an old woman with "exfoliative dermatitis" involving the whole skin surface including the face. The eruption was resistant to topical and systemic steroids. Histological evaluation demonstrated crusted scabies. *Lower panel* illustrates an old woman with recent onset psoriasis erythroderma

not preceded by a limited eruption but instead becomes generalized soon after the onset.

Of the three most common causes of exfoliative erythroderma (psoriasis, PRP, and atopic dermatitis), PRP erythroderma is the most likely to develop over a short period of time, generally a few weeks; while patients with exfoliative erythroderma secondary to psoriasis or atopic dermatitis generally have the disorder for several years prior to dissemination.

Predisposition to generalized crusted (Norwegian) scabies includes prolonged treatment with steroids and immunosuppression. In endemic areas (fogo selvagem) and untreated severe sporadic cases of PF, patients may present with generalized exfoliation instead of shallow erosions.

Patients with drug-induced exfoliative erythroderma generally present several days to three weeks following the initiation of the offending medication, which is often a medication prescribed for seizures, commonly Dilantin.

Clinical Findings

Although all of the above disorders result in overlapping and sometimes indistinguishable clinical morphology of exfoliative erythroderma, specific clinical findings in addition to history are often helpful in making a diagnosis.

For example, acute onset of a generalized eruption with fine scaling and/or desquamation following the intake of a potentially offending medication such as Dilantin would strongly point to the diagnosis of drug-induced exfoliative erythroderma, also known as *drug hypersensitivity syndrome* due to the frequent association with systemic manifestations such as lymphadenopathy and systemic eosinophilia.

Severe, prolonged itching in the face of topical and may be systemic steroids is a strong clue to the diagnosis of *crusted scabies*. Involvement of the genitalia and finger webs is a strong clue.

In the rare presentation of *PF* as exfoliative erythroderma, shallow erosions and crusting are often evident upon close inspection.

The characteristic waxy palmo-plantar involvement in *PRP*, frequently associated with "islands of sparing" and salmon color, makes the diagnosis easy.

Most patients with *psoriasis* erythroderma have history of previous psoriasis. Progression into erythroderma often follows withdrawal of systemic steroids or, less frequently, biologic agents. Extremely rarely, erythroderma may be the initial presentation of psoriasis. The diagnosis of these cases may be difficult. Supportive evidence may include strong family history, characteristic nail findings, silvery scale, and sometimes remote personal history of psoriasis.

Similarly, exfoliative erythroderma secondary to *atopic dermatitis* usually occurs in patients who have long-standing history of dermatitis, often with lichenification.

Exfoliative erythroderma secondary to *Sezary syndrome* often develops rather rapidly (over a few to several weeks). Itching may be severe and peripheral lymph nodes may be palpable. Patients often have rapid thinning of scalp hair and ectropion. This presentation should be differentiated from erythrodermic mycosis fungoides (MF). Stage IB mycosis fungoides consists of patches that involve more than 10 % of the skin surface. Infrequently, patients may have total or near-total skin involvement. These patients have a much better prognosis compared to those with Sezary syndrome.

How Helpful Is the Pathology?

At least moderately ++

Histological Findings

Some studies suggest that when a skin disorder becomes erythrodermic, it loses some or many of its histological characteristics. The degree to which histological characteristics are lost is highly variable, making it generally more difficult for the pathologist to render an accurate diagnosis.

It is recommended that two or more long "shave" biopsy specimens be obtained for the histological evaluation of patients with exfoliative erythroderma.

Disorders with Characteristic Histopathology

Disorders that are easy to diagnose include crusted scabies and pemphigus foliaceous (multiple mites and acantholysis, respectively). If PF is suspected and the histological findings are not diagnostic then immunofluorescence may be helpful.

Limitations of Histopathology

Dermatitis, psoriasis, PRP, and drug hypersensitivity syndrome share acanthosis, parakeratosis, and a superficial lymphocytic infiltrate. Differentiating among them is not always easy, especially if only one biopsy is submitted.

Findings that may favor dermatitis include spongiosis and serous crust, as well as lichenification. Findings that may favor PRP include a dilated follicular infundibulum filled with keratin, and parakeratosis alternating with orthokeratosis in both the horizontal and perpendicular planes in the stratum corneum.

Although collections of neutrophils in the stratum corneum are characteristic of psoriasis, the presence of neutrophils in patients with exfoliative erythroderma is not as diagnostic and may represent secondary bacterial colonization. Erythrodermic psoriasis may also reveal spongiosis. Features that may support the diagnosis of psoriasis are loss of the granular layer, regular epidermal hyperplasia, and dilated tortuous capillaries.

The diagnosis of cutaneous T-cell lymphoma (SS or MF) is based on the presence of small and medium-sized lymphocytes with halos in the epidermis. Sezary syndrome and erythrodermic MF, however, may both have spongiosis that may mask or overshadow the atypical lymphocytes. Clinical pathological correlation is highly essential and further biopsies may be needed. Molecular testing for T cell clonality may be needed.

Conclusions

In the evaluation of patients who are present with exfoliative erythroderma, history is extremely helpful while histological evaluation may be only moderately helpful. Multiple biopsies are often needed.

Chapter 27
Generalized Pruritus

Figure 27.1 illustrates two patients with two of the disorders discussed in this chapter.

Case A middle-aged or elderly person presents with a several month history of generalized pruritus. Examination reveals unremarkable skin or scattered excoriations among otherwise unremarkable skin.

The clinical presentation of generalized pruritus is one of the more challenging clinical presentations in dermatology. It may be due to subclinical or very mild primary dermatologic disorder, and rarely may be the initial presentation of an internal hematologic malignancy or other systemic disorder.

The differential diagnosis includes

- Mild or subclinical primary skin disorder such as
  - xerosis
  - infestation
  - dermographism
  - pemphigoid presenting as generalized pruritus, AND

- Systemic disorders such as
  - hematological disorders and malignancies
  - endocrine disorders
  - renal failure
  - hepatic failure and disorders
  - psychiatric disorders.

The main responsibility of the dermatologist is to determine which of the two disease groups does the patient's complaint belong to, hence, which patient requires an extensive and expensive systemic evaluation that may be associated with anxiety by the patient and the family.

D. F. Mutasim, *Practical Skin Pathology*, DOI 10.1007/978-3-319-14729-1_27

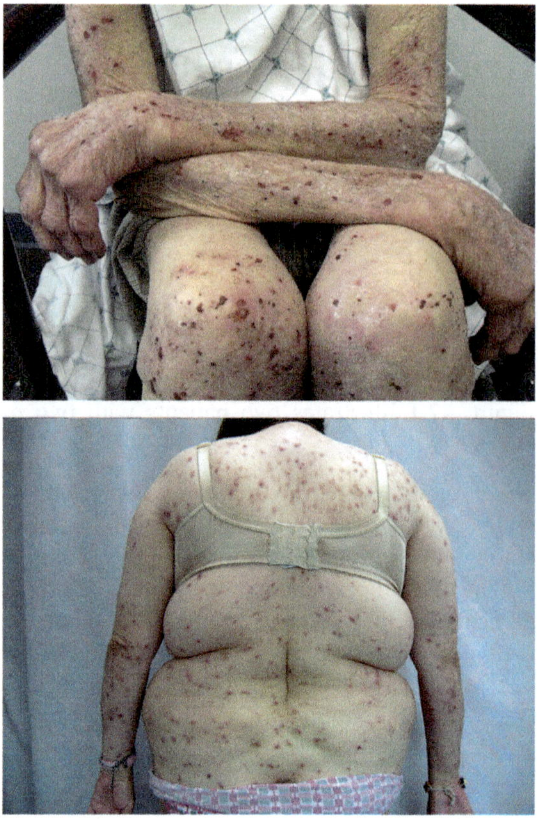

Fig. 27.1 *Upper panel* demonstrates an old woman with long history of generalized pruritus suspected to be psychogenic. Direct immunofluorescence examination confirmed the diagnosis of pemphigoid presenting as generalized pruritus. *Lower panel* demonstrates a young woman with posttraumatic stress disorders who has generalized pruritus and psychogenic excoriations

Clinical Clues

Generalized Pruritus Secondary to Dermatologic Disorders

The clinical presentation of *xerosis* is variable. Dry skin may appear ashy especially in dark-skinned individuals without being necessarily rough or obviously scaly. Sweat and/or OTC creams and lotions may also mask the abnormal appearance of the horny layer upon physical examination. Extreme dryness may lead to various clinical presentations of dermatitis, foremost among them are "cumulative insults irritant dermatitis" most often seen on the hands, and "asteatotic dermatitis" or "eczema craquele," more often seen over the lower legs, more commonly in the elderly.

In some cases in which subclinical dryness may be the cause of generalized pruritus, it is wise to treat the patient for xerosis and reevaluate in few weeks.

Subclinical infestation by scabies or pediculosis corporis may cause generalized pruritus with minimal or no physical findings. In my experience, "invisible scabies" may occur due to the use of topical steroids (which suppress the inflammatory response; hence, the clinical manifestations of the infestation), very early in the course of the infestation or in individuals who shower frequently and scrub their skin aggressively.

A possible clue to the diagnosis of subclinical scabies is the examination of the genital region, especially in males. The presence of a rare papule is often greatly rewarding. Other clues include having scabies, or simply itching in household members or sexual partners. The index of suspicion should be higher in individuals who may be exposed to patients with scabies such as in nursing homes and other crowded institutions.

Generalized dermographism presents as generalized pruritus without lesions. Some patients volunteer the observation that scratching the skin results in swelling. Whether patients with generalized pruritus offer that information or not, attempting to induce dermographism in the office may be highly rewarding in some cases. However, one should not fall into the trap of making the diagnosis of dermographism in every patient whose skin responds with redness and swelling. Some individuals may demonstrate dermographism that is evident on testing but that is not the cause of their pruritus. If a patient's generalized pruritus does not respond very well to the treatment of dermographism, then further search into the possible etiology is indicated.

"*Pemphigoid presenting as generalized pruritus*" is not as rare as initially thought. Recent data suggests that it may be common, especially in the elderly. The exact incidence compared to the bullous presentation of pemphigoid is not known. I have cared for six or seven elderly and old patients with pemphigoid presenting only with pruritus with or without excoriations. I also read a few positive direct immunofluorescence tests on other patients with pruritus with excoriations only. Some were suspected to have dermatitis herpetiformis. Unlike the majority of cases of bullous pemphigoid, skin folds are not necessarily favored in patients with pemphigoid presenting as generalized pruritus.

Confirming this disorder requires direct immunofluorescence of a biopsy specimen. This may be a shave or punch biopsy from a site that is pruritic. Whether one biopsy is enough to confirm or exclude pemphigoid in patients with this clinical presentation is not known. If no other etiology for generalized pruritus has been found and one immunofluorescence test is nonspecific or negative, another from a different site may help confirm the diagnosis. Indirect immunofluorescence is not as reliable and should not be used as a substitute for direct immunofluorescence. The response of these patients to systemic steroids, usually in small doses, or super potent topical steroids is often dramatic.

Patients with generalized itchy papules/*hypersensitivity reaction* may excoriate all lesions leaving no primary lesions for the practitioner to suspect the diagnosis. History of primary papules or photographic documentation of papules by the patient should alert the practitioner to search for a primary lesion to perform a biopsy for histological evaluation. In my experience, a few patients who have unhappily carried the diagnosis of "psychogenic pruritus with excoriation" and kept searching for another diagnosis indeed had severely excoriated hypersensitivity reaction/prurigo simplex or reaction to insect bites.

Generalized Pruritus Secondary to Systemic Disorders

Generalized pruritus may be secondary to hematologic disorders, especially Hodgkin's lymphoma, polycythemia vera, anemia, and rarely might be the presenting sign of Sezary syndrome. It may also be secondary to metabolic disorders, such as renal failure and liver failure; and endocrine disorders such as thyroid disease and possibly diabetes. The diagnosis of renal and/or liver failure is usually known at the time of presentation, while the diagnosis of the hematologic disorder or thyroid disease may not be known.

Psychiatric disorders are known to be associated with multiple skin manifestations including generalized pruritus referred to as "psychogenic pruritus." One should be cautious in making this diagnosis as it precludes further evaluation and labels the patient in a manner that may not be easily defensible. Unless the clinical evidence for a psychogenic cause is great, patients with generalized pruritus with negative systemic evaluation, and in whom a subclinical skin disorder has been excluded may be told to have primary or idiopathic pruritus.

How Helpful Is the Pathology?

Slightly +

Except for confirming the diagnosis of pemphigoid by immunofluorescence, a biopsy specimen is of little value in the evaluation of patients with generalized pruritus.

Historical Clues

In the absence of clinical findings, history acquires great importance. Although itching is subjective and patients may vary in their attempt to evaluate it on an objective scale, with proper prompting by the dermatologist, most patients are able to grade the severity of their pruritus on at least a three-point scale (mild, moderate, severe) and many on a five- or ten-point scale.

Severe or unbearable pruritus, especially if it is rapidly progressive, is generally a sign of an internal disorder, often a hematologic malignancy. Unlike patients with severe generalized pruritus secondary to end-stage liver or end-stage kidney disease, in whom the underlying diagnosis is known, generalized pruritus may be the presenting manifestation of a hematologic malignancy thus the importance of dermatologic consultation.

Of the causes of generalized pruritus that are due to a primary subclinical skin disorder, the itching in subclinical scabies may also be severe or unbearable. Itching secondary to dermographism, xerosis, and subclinical pemphigoid is generally moderate in severity.

Conclusions

Patients who present with generalized pruritus are among the more challenging cases faced by the dermatologist. Detailed history, examination, and review of systems and medical history are all important in arriving at the diagnosis. Histopathology is helpful only rarely.

Chapter 28
Photo-Eruptions

Figure 28.1 illustrates two patients with two of the disorders discussed in this chapter.

Introduction—Pathways to Photosensitivity

The way by which light plays a role in photo-eruptions varies among disorders. Some eruptions such as *solar urticaria, polymorphous light eruption (PMLE), photo-contact dermatitis, and photo-drug eruption,* require a specific dose of ultraviolet exposure in order to *induce* the eruption. Without exposure to the necessary dose of ultraviolet light, patients may not manifest their disorder.

Other disorders, such as *lupus erythematosus (LE) and dermatomyositis (DM)* usually occur without a specific occasion of light exposure but are often *exacerbated* by ultraviolet light exposure. Occasionally, however, the first manifestation of lupus (especially subacute lupus) or dermatomyositis may follow an episode of excessive sun exposure.

Finally some disorders, specifically some forms of *porphyria,* which result from excessive levels of porphyrin in the skin, require chronically sun-exposed or *sun-damaged skin* in order to manifest skin lesions. Although the levels of porphyrin are similar throughout the skin, the manifestations of the disorder are limited to chronically sun-exposed sites. Ultraviolet light is required for interaction with porphyrin in the skin in order to result in a cascade of events that cause skin fragility and easy trauma-induced blistering.

Chronic actinic dermatitis (CAD) is somewhat unique. Some patients have pre-existing dermatitis that is exacerbated by light (so-called photosensitive eczema). Others have an eruption that is initiated by light exposure either in the presence of a photo-sensitizing drug, but that persists after discontinuing the medication (persistent light reaction) or without a medication (actinic reticuloid).

D. F. Mutasim, *Practical Skin Pathology,* DOI 10.1007/978-3-319-14729-1_28

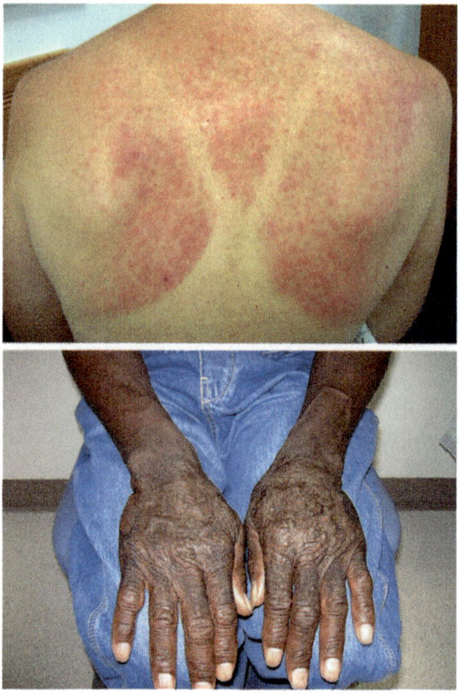

Fig. 28.1 *Upper panel* illustrates a young woman who reported short-lived eruption secondary to sun exposure. She was asked to reproduce the eruption before the next visit. Histological examination confirmed the diagnosis of acute photosensitive lupus erythematosus. *Lower panel* illustrates an elderly African American man with chronic actinic dermatitis secondary to persistent light reaction due to hydrochlorothiazide. The patient had involvement of the face and posterior neck as well. His UVA minimum erythema dose was 4 J

History

In patients suspected to have a photosensitive disorder, history is extremely useful.

Is the patient aware of a relation between sun exposure and skin lesions? If so, how long is the incubation period between exposure and onset of lesions? What is the morphology of the lesions? How long is the duration of lesions if sun exposure is discontinued? What happens with continued light exposure?

In general, all patients with solar urticaria and erythropoeitic protoporphyria (EPP) and most patients with polymorphous light eruption (PMLE) are highly aware of the connection between the skin lesions and sun exposure. Patients with solar urticaria develop hives a few minutes following regular sun exposure. Patients with PMLE get lesions one to few days following excessive sun exposure. Patients with EPP, often children, get burning and painful lesions within seconds or minutes of sun exposure.

Patients with porphyria cutanea tarda (PCT) and pseudo-PCT are generally less aware of a relationship of their disorder to sun exposure. When questioned, they may report that their disorder is more active during summertime, but rarely report a specific exposure as causing their blisters.

That is due to the fact that the direct cause of blistering in PCT and pseudo-PCT is minor trauma and not an episode of sun exposure. Chronic exposure to light is necessary for photoactivation of porphyrin that results in skin fragility; hence, easy blistering with minor trauma; thus, the clinical similarity between PCT and EBA type I (in which antibodies against the basement membrane attack collagen VII molecules in anchoring fibrils of the sublamina densa of the basement membrane, resulting in skin fragility and easy blistering).

Patients with PMLE are well known to develop the phenomenon of hardening with repeated light exposure. This is the foundation of treating PMLE patients with phototherapy.

Clinical Findings

Just as medications cause a multitude of skin eruptions, so does sunlight. Photosensitive eruptions may present with hives (solar urticaria), smooth papules-nodules-plaques (PMLE), vesicles-bullae (PCT, pseudo-PCT, EPP, severe phototoxic drug eruption), red patches-plaques (LE and DM), spongiotic dermatitis (drug-induced photodermatitis), and lichenoid dermatitis (lichenoid photodrug eruption).

Histological Findings

There are as many histological types of photo-eruptions as there are clinical types. Just as drug eruptions, photo-eruptions belong to several morphological categories; hence, multiple histological patterns, including spongiotic, lichenoid interface, subepidermal vesicle, dermal lymphocytic infiltrate, and urticaria may be seen. Just as drug etiology can rarely be determined by histopathology, ultraviolet light etiology can rarely be inferred from histological findings alone. For example, a noninflammatory subepidermal vesicle may either be EBA or PCT/pseudo-PCT, and spongiotic dermatitis can be due to eczematous dermatitis or photodermatitis (photodrug eruption).

Some Subtle histological features have been proposed to favor light etiology; for example, dyskeratosis or sunburn cells and extension of the infiltrate from the papillary dermis into the reticular dermis), but their power of prediction is weak. The best way to confirm photosensitivity is phototesting, where available.

Conclusions

Photodermatoses are a morphologically heterogeneous group of disorders. History is extremely important and histology is of little value, except in confirming the clinical morphology of the disorder.

Chapter 29
Hypopigmented Patches

Figure 29.1 illustrates two patients with two of the disorders discussed in this chapter.

Case A patient presents with a diffuse eruption consisting of multiple hypopigmented macules.

A solitary hypopigmented patch often represents nevus hypopigmentosus or depigmentosus, or nevus anemicus (which is not truly hypopigmented but instead pale due to vasoconstriction). Occasionally, intradermal or intra-articular steroid injection may result in hypopigmentation without appreciable atrophy. These disorders will not be addressed here.

Clinical differential diagnosis includes

- pityriasis alba (P. Alba)
- mycosis fungoides (MF)
- sarcoidosis
- early vitiligo
- progressive macular hypomelanosis (PMH)
- tinea versicolor (TV), and
- lichen sclerosis (LS).

It is important to note that lesions of LS are not truly hypopigmented, but appear whitish secondary to the aberrant physical properties of the abnormal papillary dermis, just as lesions of atrophoderma appear brownish without having increased pigmentation.

These disorders vary in their pathophysiology from mild inflammation (P. Alba) to autoimmune (vitiligo) to lymphoma (MF) and a granulomatous disorder (sarcoidosis).

Clinical Clues

Clinical clues are moderately helpful in the differential diagnosis.

D. F. Mutasim, *Practical Skin Pathology*, DOI 10.1007/978-3-319-14729-1_29

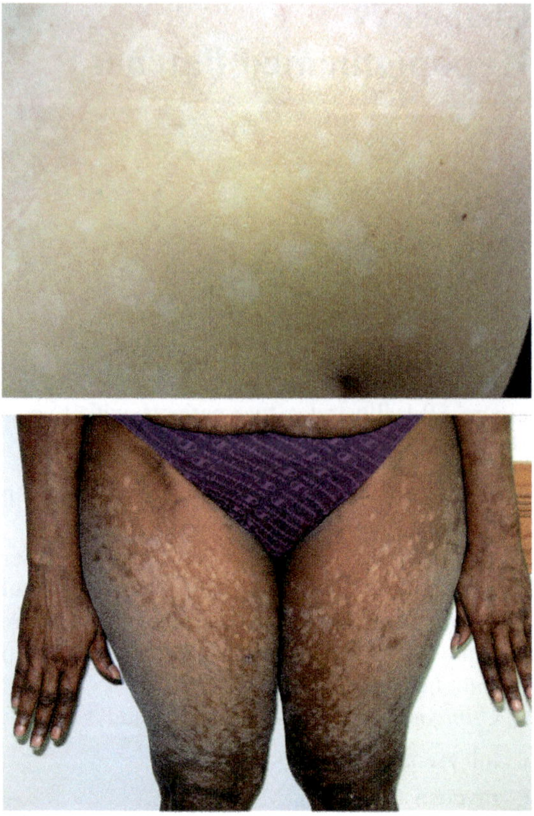

Fig. 29.1 *Upper panel* demonstrates a young woman with progressive macular hypomelanosis. Note the multiple smooth hypopigmented macules. *Lower panel* demonstrated an African–American woman with extensive minimally finely scaly hypopigmented macules of mycosis fungoides

Morphological Clues

All disorders in this group present with lesions that are *well defined*, except P. Alba and PMH, in which lesions are ill-defined. Although all the above disorders appear macular, some lesions of LS and sarcoidosis may be *palpable*.

Early vitiligo is strongly favored if some of the lesions are *depigmented* or if mucous membranes are involved.

Faint erythema may be seen in some lesions of MF, sarcoidosis, and early vitiligo.

In addition to whitish macules that represent old lesions, patients with active LS have lesions that show *telangiectasia* and pinpoint *petechiae*, as well as rough, slightly scaly surface with minute keratotic plugs (in follicular and eccrine ostia).

Other Clues

Young age (childhood and early adulthood) and history of atopy may favor P. Alba. Most other disorders occur in older adults.

Treated and sometimes untreated TV often results in hypopigmentation, especially in the face of chronic sun exposure, which results in tanning of adjacent uninvolved skin. The distribution of lesions and their pattern is often easily recognized as TV.

The presence of lesions on *genital* skin raises suspicion for LS and vitiligo.

How Helpful Is the Pathology?

At least moderately++

Histological Clues

The histological findings of *sarcoidosis* and *LS* are highly characteristic, well known, and easily recognizable. The so-called naked granulomas are characteristic of sarcoidosis in the absence of organisms or foreign bodies. Edema and hyalinization of an expanded papillary dermis are characteristic of LS. The histological findings in the remaining disorders in this group are generally mild and may be subtle, so a specific diagnosis may not be always possible.

The organisms in *TV* may be recognized by standard microscopy due to their abundance in the stratum corneum, or by special fungal stain. The findings in hypopigmented *MF* are similar to those in patch-stage MF with other clinical presentations, that is, single or clustered lymphocytes with halos predominantly in the epidermal basal layer with no or minimal spongiosis.

The histological findings of P. Alba, PMH, and early vitiligo are not diagnostic and differentiation among the three disorders is not always possible by histopathology.

P. Alba is characterized by mild focal parakeratosis, mild focal spongiosis, and a mild superficial lymphocytic infiltrate; in other words, mild spongiotic dermatitis. The differential diagnosis of mild spongiotic dermatitis is wide, however, and includes digitate dermatosis (small plaque parapsoriasis) and mild eczematous dermatitis. Clinical correlation is extremely important in confirming the diagnosis of P. Alba.

Similarly, the diagnosis of early hypopigmented *vitiligo* requires clinical correlation. The findings in early or hypopigmented vitiligo consist of decreased epidermal pigmentation and possibly a mild superficial lymphocytic infiltrate with or without a few melanophages. The decreased epidermal pigmentation may not be appreciated if the pathologist does not have a biopsy specimen from adjacent normal pigmented skin to compare with, and the infiltrate may be too mild to appreciate or sometimes absent.

The most commonly submitted differential diagnosis for disorders in this section is early vitiligo versus hypopigmented MF versus hypopigmented sarcoidosis. The lack of findings to support sarcoidosis and MF may suffice for the pathologist to agree with the clinical suspicion of vitiligo. An immunohistochemical study using antibodies to melanocytes (such as S 100 protein and MITF) is often helpful by confirming loss of or a decreased number of basal melanocytes. It is strongly suggested that two biopsy specimens are submitted in patients suspected to have early or hypopigmented vitiligo. Alternatively, one marked incisional biopsy specimen, including the border and adjacent normal appearing skin, may suffice.

There are no characteristic histological findings in *PMH* besides decreased pigmentation of the epidermis. The diagnosis is often made clinically and by excluding other hypopigmentary disorders. PMH favors the trunk of females and individuals of color and presents with discrete and confluent ill-defined hypopigmented macules. Some authors propose that cases previously diagnosed as generalized P. Alba actually represent PMH. The exact cause and best treatment for PMH is not known. It has been proposed that normal bacterial flora of the hair follicle may be responsible.

Conclusions

The differential diagnosis of hypopigmented macules or patches is wide. Few disorders are histologically characteristic (sarcoidosis, LS, and MF), while others require clinicopathological correlation.

Chapter 30
Pigmented Patches

Figure 30.1 illustrates two patients with two of the disorders discussed in this chapter.

Case A patient presents with multiple, acquired, smooth brownish patches.

Lesions are acquired, so congenital pigmentation, such as café au lait spots, are excluded; lesions are smooth and nonpalpable; hence, chronic hyperpigmented disorders, such as dermatitis and hyperpigmented mycosis fungoides (MF), are excluded.

The clinical differential diagnosis includes

- erythema dyschromicum perstans EDP/ashy dermatosis
- drug deposition
- macular amyloidosis
- melasma
- lymphocytic macular arteritis (LMA)
- post-fixed drug eruption (FDE)
- phytophotodermatitis, and
- atrophoderma.

Although lesions of *atrophoderma* appear brown, there is no increased pigmentation, unlike the other disorders in this group. The brownish appearance in atrophoderma is due to the way light is reflected from skin with atrophic dermis. The characteristic depressed border is easily detected, especially by using incident lighting. Without appreciating the border, a lesion of atrophoderma may be mistaken for macular hyperpigmentation.

Clinical Clues

1. Clues based on patients' ethnicity

Both melasma and macular amyloidosis are more common among individuals of Middle Eastern and Asian background. EDP/ashy dermatosis is common in

D. F. Mutasim, *Practical Skin Pathology*, DOI 10.1007/978-3-319-14729-1_30

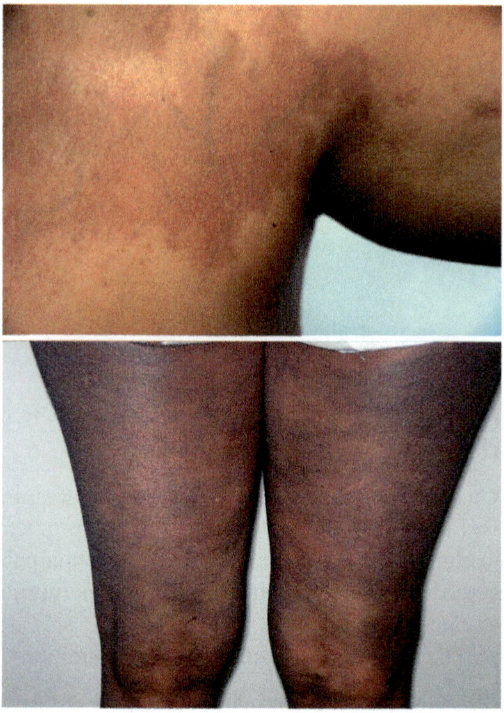

Fig. 30.1 *Upper panel* reveals a young woman with type IV skin and confluent brownish, depressed, smooth patches characteristic of atrophoderma. *Lower panel* reveals a woman with type V skin and multiple ashy smooth macules, characteristic of ashy dermatosis

individuals of color such as Latin Americans. LMA predominantly affects individuals of color that include Middle Eastern, African American, and Asian.

2. Clues based on location

Melasma invariably involves the face and rarely the upper extremities as well. Macular amyloidosis almost always involves the upper back, and often is limited to the upper back.

Deposition of drug or drug metabolites, such as hydroxychloroquine, amiodarone, and imipramine, favors the sun-exposed skin. Hydroxychloroquine and chloroquine pigmentation favors the lower legs, and to a lesser degree to the arms. Chlorpromazine pigmentation favors the face and nail beds in addition to the extremities. Minocycline produces three types of pigmentation: deep blue in acne scars, diffuse brown on sun-exposed skin, and blue–grey on the lower legs.

Similarly, LMA invariably involves the lower legs and occasionally the thighs. Pigmentation secondary to phytophotodermatitis is predominantly seen over sun-exposed skin. Fixed drug eruption favors mucocutaneous areas such as the lips and genitalia. Lesions of ashy dermatosis (often used synonymously with erythema dyschromicum perstans (EDP)) favor the trunk but only slightly.

3. Clues based on morphology

Lesions of FDE are uniformly round or near-round, as are the lesions of EDP and LMA. Lesions of melasma are extremely symmetrical and are irregularly shaped, and those of phytophotodermatitis are figurate.

Lesions of FDE, LMA, EDP, atrophoderma, and melasma are well defined. Lesions of macular amyloidosis are ill-defined, consisting of confluent punctate tiny macules extending gradually outwardly, often in a rippled pattern.

The color is brown in all the above disorders except EDP/ashy dermatosis (in which it is characteristically grayish) and some drug deposition. Pigmentation secondary to minocycline, imipramine, and amiodarone has a bluish–gray hue. Chlorpromazine facial pigmentation is purplish, while antimalarial pigmentation like that of LMA is primarily brownish.

A few patients with EDP/ashy dermatosis may have associated active lesions appearing as pink or red annular or serpiginous macules with a tiny thread-like border. Such lesions may be seen alone or at the outer margin of ashy macules, indicating continued disease activity at the lesion borders.

Course

Lesions in all the above disorders are chronic, generally persistent, and resistant to treatment.

How Helpful Is the Pathology?

Moderately + +

Histological findings

EDP/ashy dermatosis, macular amyloidosis, melasma, post-FDE, and phytophotodermatitis are all characterized by so-called pigment incontinence or dermal melanosis. Melanophages abound in the papillary and superficial reticular dermis. Some melanin brown granules may also be seen outside macrophages in the same region.

The relationship between *EDP* and ashy dermatosis has been debated. Some authors use the two terms interchangeably while others propose that they are two separate but related disorders; yet others use the term EDP to refer to the short-lived inflammatory disease process whose end result is grayish pigmentation; hence, "ashy dermatosis." In the original paper describing EDP, the authors used the term ashy dermatosis and introduced the term EDP to differentiate their disorder from other forms of erythema perstans (EP) that are not associated with pigmentation.

The inflammatory phase of EDP/ashy dermatosis is characterized by basal vacuolization and a generally mild lymphocytic infiltrate in the basal layer and around capillaries in the papillary dermis. Similar but milder findings may be seen in ashy macules without erythema. Similar histological findings are seen in the involuting lesions of other disorders, which are characterized by lichenoid interface dermatitis, especially LP; hence, the proposition by some that EDP/ashy dermatosis to be considered a variant of LP. The clinical presentation, however, is so unique that the term is best retained.

Macular amyloidosis is a clinical diagnosis that rarely requires histological confirmation. Sections may seem unremarkable at scanning magnification or some melanophages may be clearly evident. Further examination often yields hints of keratinocyte dyskeratosis, minute foci of indistinct basal cells beneath which tiny amounts of homogeneous pink material, often admixed with few melanophages, are identified. In some cases, the amyloid deposits are more abundant; then, one often sees two adjacent rete clawed inward as if to hug or engulf the amyloid material, a finding more easily seen in lichen or papular amyloidosis.

Melasma is also a clinical diagnosis. Histopathology is sometimes obtained in order to assess if the increased pigmentation is epidermal, dermal, or combined, and to assess the depth of melanin in the dermis prior to laser treatment.

Pigmentation secondary to medication has variable histological findings. In general, pigment granules are seen inside and outside of macrophages in the dermis. Some or all granules have staining characteristics of melanin. The exact molecular nature of the granules is not known.

Conclusions

The differential diagnosis of pigmented patches is wide and requires a detailed dermatological and medical history including medications. A biopsy specimen may sometimes be helpful.

Chapter 31
Red Smooth Patches

Figure 31.1 illustrates two patients with two of the disorders discussed in this chapter.

Case A patient presents with a few to several weeks' history of confluent red smooth macules and patches. The onset may be acute or insidious and favors photo-exposed sites. This presentation is exclusive of the patients with total skin erythroderma, in whom the differential diagnosis is different (see Chap. 26 on exfoliative erythroderma).

Clinical Differential Diagnosis Depends on the onset and duration of the eruption. If acute and short-lived, then the patient is likely to have morbilliform drug eruption or exanthem (not addressed here); and if subacute to chronic, then,

- dermatomyositis, DM
- photosensitive rash of systemic lupus erythematosus, SLE
- photosensitive dermatitis/photo-drug eruption, and
- subacute cutaneous lupus erythematosus, SCLE.

Clinical Clues

Lesions of *SCLE* are almost always discrete (annular polycyclic or psoriasiform, and rarely pityriasiform), unlike those of DM and the photosensitive rash of SLE, which are often diffuse. However, SCLE has been described as presenting in a diffuse manner as exfoliative erythroderma, even with bullae and TEN-like presentation. In my experience, this occurs in patients who are extremely photosensitive, following excessive sun exposure, resulting in the first episode of SCLE in an unsuspecting patient. Few patients with SCLE may have mild SLE.

D. F. Mutasim, *Practical Skin Pathology*, DOI 10.1007/978-3-319-14729-1_31

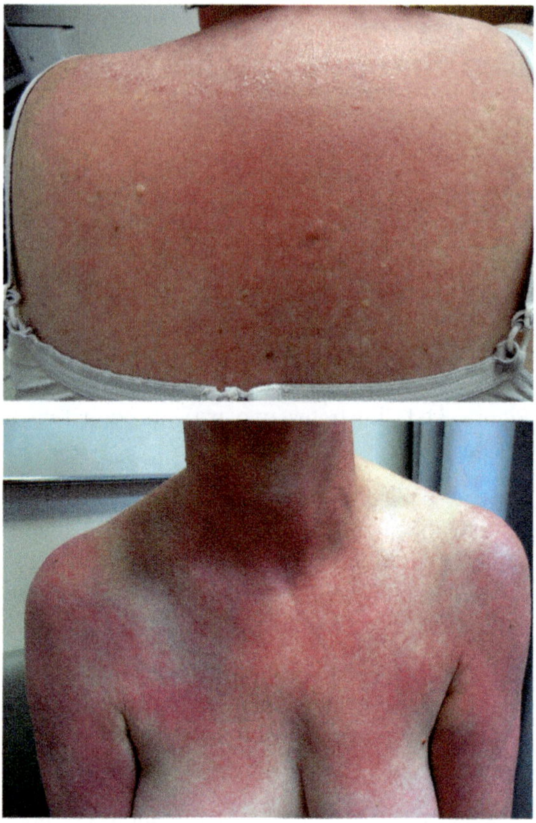

Fig. 31.1 *Upper panel* reveals a young woman who presented with acute generalized photo-induced erythema, acral vasculopathy of the fingers and toes, oral erosions, and proteinuria, all features of systemic lupus erythematosus. *Lower panel* reveals an elderly woman with dermatomyositis. Note the *brightly red* erythema sparing sun-protected sites

The first episode of the photosensitive eruption in patients with undiagnosed *SLE* or *DM* may appear similar to and be confused with photosensitive drug eruption. Involvement of the eyelids with edema and purplish erythema is a characteristic of DM, while erythema, in the butterfly distribution, in the absence of eyelid involvement strongly favors SLE.

Photosensitive Drug Eruption May be toxic (often seen in dermatology with doxycycline) or allergic (a long list of medications) with great overlap and imperfect distinction (hence, the more inclusive term "photosensitive drug eruption" is preferred). Phototoxic reaction mimics sunburn and is greatly photo-distributed. Photoallergic reaction mimics spongiotic dermatitis, usually subacute, both clinically and histologically. Some photosensitive eruptions are histologically and clinically lichenoid. These are more often papular.

How Helpful Is the Pathology?

Not helpful +

Histological Findings

The combination of basal vacuolization, mild superficial and deep lymphocytic infiltrate, usually with increased dermal mucin, is characteristic of DM, SCLE and the acute photo-induced rash of SLE. If the photoeruption of SLE becomes chronic and persistent, it may acquire hyperkeratosis, dilated follicles, and a more prominent perifollicular infiltrate, reminiscent of discoid LE.

Spongiotic and lichenoid photo-drug eruptions mimic spongiotic dermatitis and lichenoid interface dermatitis. There are no specific features that indicate photosensitivity as a cause in either pattern of other causes. Some authors have proposed that the infiltrate in photosensitive dermatitis is likely to extend below the papillary dermis. This is however not reliable. Phototesting remains the gold standard for proving photosensitivity. Most patients with drug-induced photosensitivity are highly sensitive to Ultraviolet A (UVA). Not only is the minimal erythema dose markedly decreased but also UVA irradiation often reproduces the lesions.

How About Direct Immunofluorescence (DIF)?

DIF is also not helpful.

I have evaluated hundreds of direct immunofluorescence (DIF) biopsy specimens over the past 30 years from dermatologists asking to differentiate between DM and LE. These requests are often made after receiving a pathology report that indicates that the differential diagnosis is DM and LE. Some pathologists then recommend that the clinician obtain DIF in order to differentiate between the two disorders. Rarely has the test been helpful. In most cases, DIF is negative or mild and nonspecific even in cases that later prove to be LE. DIF is most likely to be positive in chronic discoid lesions and is frequently negative in acute and subacute lesions of lupus.

The literature quotes a figure of around 70 % positivity of DIF in SCLE and a similar figure in DM. While it is true that there are immune deposits at the dermo–epidermal junction in both DM and SCLE, the intensity is mild and the pattern is often not continuous along the dermo–epidermal junction; hence, the diagnosis of DM and LE cannot be confirmed nor excluded. A rare lesion of SCLE may demonstrate granular immunoglobulin deposits within basal and to a lesser degree suprabasal keratinocytes cytoplasm and nuclei. This pattern was initially reported in patients with mixed connective tissue disease with high titers of anti-RNP antibodies but later found in other patients with other connective tissue diseases along with other antinuclear antibodies.

In SLE patients with anti-double stranded DNA antibodies and generally renal disease DIF of lesional skin, and sometimes normal skin is frequently positive. There is an obvious deposition of immunoglobulins and complement in the form of a band (thus the historical term Lupus band test) of granular and/or of homogeneous material.

How About Blood Tests?

Serologic testing is very useful in the differentiation of the above disorders.

The antinuclear antibody test (ANA), whether by traditional immunofluorescence or by the more recent quantitative ANA-Direct test, is positive in 80–85 % in DM and SCLE and 100 % in SLE.

The pattern is speckled in DM and SCLE, and homogeneous and or peripheral/rim in SLE. Disease-specific antibodies in SCLE are SSA/Ro and SSB/La, while there are multiple autoantibodies in DM and SLE.

Conclusions

In the evaluation of red, smooth patches, a biopsy specimen is useful to differentiate between vacuolar interface dermatitis of DM, SLE, and SCLE on one side and photodermatitis, spongiotic, or lichenoid on the other. Serological testing is extremely helpful. Phototesting may be necessary occasionally.

Chapter 32
Red Scaly Patches

Figure 32.1 illustrates two patients with two of the disorders discussed in this chapter.

Case A patient presents with a few months to a few years' history of an eruption of discrete and confluent scaly red patches—not lichenified, not hyperkeratotic, not erosive, with no pustules, and no crust.

Clinical differential diagnosis includes

- thin psoriasis
- pityriasis rubra pilaris (PRP)
- mycosis fungoides (MF)
- MF-like drug eruption
- subacute dermatitis, and
- parapsoriasis.

The latter disorder will be discussed separately at the end of this chapter due to its more complex nosology.

Clinical Clues

Psoriasis and *PRP* may share clinical and histological features. Both disorders are striking in their redness. The other five disorders are not. Early lesions of psoriasis and PRP are rather easy to differentiate but the two disorders may be difficult to distinguish clinically and histologically when both are advancing to or are in a state of erythroderma.

Rarely, an eruption of scaly, large patches follows interferon injections for hepatitis in a patient with no prior history of psoriasis. It looks clinically and histologically like psoriasis, but usually subsides with discontinuation of interferon. Whether it is true psoriasis or not, is not clear.

D. F. Mutasim, *Practical Skin Pathology*, DOI 10.1007/978-3-319-14729-1_32

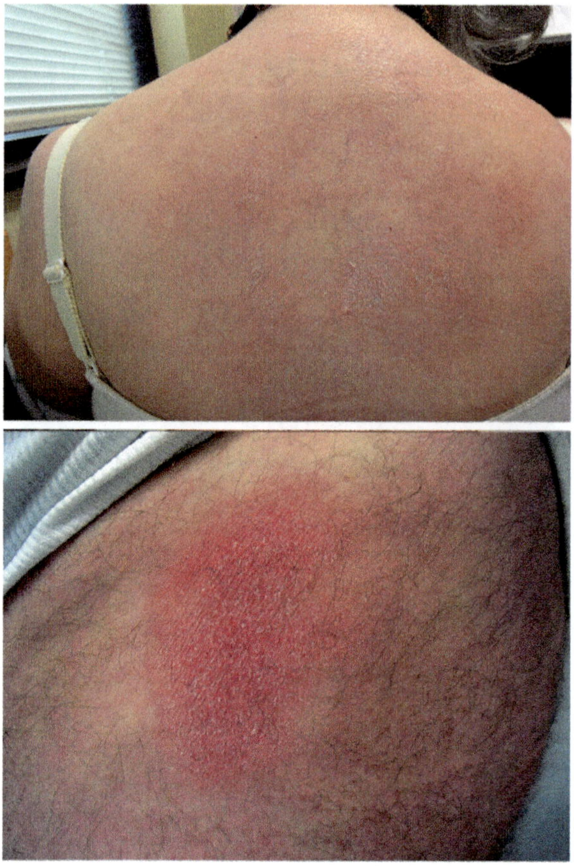

Fig. 32.1 *Upper panel* demonstrates a patient with scattered slightly erythematosus finely scaling patches of lymphomatoid drug eruption, also known as mycosis fungoides-like drug eruption. *Lower panel* demonstrates an elderly man with few scattered ill-defined, oval–to-round erythematosus, fine, scaly patches of mycosis fungoides

Adult PRP, on the other hand, most often presents as a rapidly progressive eruption of papules and/or patches, invariably with islands of sparing that only rarely may disappear as PRP becomes complete erythroderma.

Patch MF has a slow onset and generally very slow progression. Patients usually have lesions for many months to few years before presenting to a dermatologist. MF is a great clinical mimicker but generally presents as poikilodermatous patches favoring flexures and skin folds, or large, thin, scaly, reddish brown patches.

MF-like drug eruption (also referred to as lymphomatoid drug eruption or drug-induced T-cell pseudolymphoma) presents to the dermatologist either as an acute drug eruption with features of subacute dermatitis that may become erythroderma and on biopsy reveals features of MF, or as an insidious eruption of faintly reddish, scaly patches that may be nondescript. The former presentation was initially described as "the anticonvulsant hypersensitivity syndrome" and related disorders.

MF-like drug eruption is rarely diagnosed clinically and may go undiagnosed histologically. With a low index of suspicion, the findings may be interpreted as consistent with drug eruption or spongiotic dermatitis.

How Helpful Is the Pathology?

Very helpful+++

Histological Findings

Patients with *dermatitis*, rarely if ever, require a biopsy for histological confirmation.

Psoriasis and *PRP* share some histological findings (acanthosis and hyper-parakeratosis), but in general may be differentiated in most cases. Neutrophils in the parakeratosis or the granular layer, significant loss of granular layer, tortuous capillaries in dermal papillae, and atrophy of the supra-papillary epidermis, all speak strongly for psoriasis. Parakeratosis alternating with orthokeratosis in both planes in the stratum corneum favor PRP.

In adult PRP, involvements of palms, soles, and scalp is almost universal and islands of sparing are common, making differentiation from erythrodermic psoriasis possible.

The finding of single or grouped lymphocytes with clear halos in the epidermis or only the basal layer with no or minimal spongiosis is diagnostic of *MF*. Early lesions of patch MF or those partially treated usually reveal subtle nondiagnostic findings.

Clues to the possible diagnosis of MF in such cases include papillary dermal fibrosis, spread of the mild perivascular infiltrate outside the immediate perivascular area almost approaching a band-like pattern, and a silent epidermis, in other words, without spongiosis, acanthosis, or significant parakeratosis. If the diagnosis is still not made, further biopsies preferably by the shave technique, are indicated.

If the diagnosis of MF still cannot be confirmed histologically, would *molecular testing for lymphocyte clonality* in a biopsy specimen *be helpful*?

Highly unlikely. The likelihood of having enough rearranged, clonal lymphocyte DNA in early MF is low. And the chance for a false-positive result in a non-MF lesion further complicates interpretation.

So What Is a Practitioner to Do? If the clinical findings are consistent with MF and no other diagnosis can be made by histopathology, then it is safe to make the diagnosis of presumed MF and act accordingly, keeping in mind that the diagnosis may become certain at a later date. If treatment is needed, one lesion may be left without treatment for observation and future biopsy.

How About MF-like Drug Eruption? This diagnosis may be suspected in cases with features that are intermediate between patch MF and subacute spongiotic dermatitis clinically and/or histologically, such as "spongiotic dermatitis with suggestion of epidermotropism" or "consistent with MF but with spongiosis."

How Is the Diagnosis of MF-like Drug Eruption Confirmed? Only by discontinuing the medication and observing involution of the eruption. But, this may take several weeks to a few months. MF-like drug eruption is unlike most other forms of drug eruption; it is not allergic/hypersensitivity, such as in acute urticaria, but instead a result of direct effect of the drug or its metabolites on the lymphocytes, as if stimulating them to migrate to the skin, reside in the epidermis, and cause lesions.

One common problem in suspecting the offending drug is that it usually is a commonly used one, such as an antihypertensive, lipid-lowering agent, oral hypoglycemic, anti-depressant, and the like.

A rare but important problem in confirming the diagnosis is that there is synergism among the many offending drugs and two drugs may need to be eliminated for the eruption to clear.

A third problem/misconception is that there is cross-over between structurally related drugs. Indeed, drugs that have different structures but a similar mechanism of action cross react. For example, a patient with an eruption due to angiotensin converting enzyme inhibitor may get a recurrence of the eruption if later given a non-chemically related angiotensin receptor blocker drug, which exerts the same effect.

Conclusions

In the evaluation of a patient with the red scaly patches, it is preferable to do two or more biopsies. Then, an accurate diagnosis is highly likely to be made.

What Is Parapsoriasis?

History and Nomenclature

Parapsoriasis was initially coined by Dr. Brocq, in 1902. In his classification of skin disorders (eczematous, lichenoid, psoriasiform, and so on), few disorders did not fit into the classification; hence, he gave them the collective term "parapsoriasis."

The term referred not to the clinical similarity of these disorders with psoriasis but instead to their similarity to psoriasis in their general lack of symptoms, chronic course, and generally poor response to then available treatments.

Dr. Brocq identified three groups of parapsoriasis based on the lesion morphology. So-called parapsoriasis *en goutte* was applied to those eruptions in which the lesions were guttate or small papules. This group included the disorders of pityriasis lichenoides previously also referred to as Mucha Habermann disease.

Parapsoriasis *en plaque* (plaque being the French word for patch or sheet) was assigned to disorders that presented with patches. Parapsoriasis *en plaque* was further divided into parapsoriasis *en plaque* small plaque type and parapsoriasis en plaque large plaque type, with lesions of the former being a few centimeters and those of the latter many centimeters in size. The two terms were replaced by "small plaque parapsoriasis" and "large plaque parapsoriasis," each also known under other names based on further morphological subclassification (digitate dermatosis, xanthoerythrodermia Perstans, parapsoriasis variegate, parakeratosis variegate, and reteform parapsoriasis).

It was realized early on that patients with large plaque parapsoriasis but not those with small plaque parapsoriasis may progress to patch-stage MF approximately 10 % of the time.

In the rest of the discussion, the term parapsoriasis is used synonymously with parapsoriasis *en plaque*.

Nosology

The nosology of the parapsoriasis remained enigmatic.

There was a significant difference in understanding parapsoriasis between dermatologists and pathologists in Europe versus those in the USA. Europeans recognized and diagnosed parapsoriasis much more frequently than Americans.

It was soon realized that the histological findings of parapsoriasis and MF overlapped. There was difficulty in clearly defining the histological differences between parapsoriasis and MF. The two disorders shared parakeratosis, minimal to no spongiosis, possible acanthosis, and a superficial lymphocytic infiltrate within a generally fibrotic papillary dermis. If significant epidermotropism of lymphocytes with halos was present, then the diagnosis of MF was rendered in both Europe and the USA. If epidermotropism was minimal, then the diagnosis of parapsoriasis was more likely to be made in Europe. In other words, few epidermotropic lymphocytes were allowed to be present in parapsoriasis by European pathologists without automatically making the diagnosis of MF.

It soon became clear that many patients with MF had variable degree of epidermotropism in different lesions, leading to interpreting some lesions as parapsoriasis and others as MF or consistent with MF. Hence, the concept of progression of parapsoriasis into MF became doubtful and the idea that parapsoriasis is a form of MF born.

The esteemed US dermatologist and dermatopathologist, A. B. Ackerman, wrote and spoke extensively that the term parapsoriasis be deleted since there were no specific defining histological characteristics for it that may not be seen also in MF. He presented arguments for his view that parapsoriasis is actually early or patch MF, and that parapsoriasis is not a precursor for MF but its first manifestation and one of many of its clinical presentations.

Whether parapsoriasis is a precursor to or is early MF is more a philosophical discussion rather than a scientifically tested hypothesis; hence, the prolonged phase of back and forth editorials on the pages of dermatology and dermatopathology journals during the 1980s and 1990s.

Finally, world-renowned European dermatologists and pathologists who have managed many patients with skin lymphomas accepted the idea that parapsoriasis is a clinical form of early or patch-stage MF. This may be one of the reasons why the apparent incidence of MF is on the rise in the past few decades.

Should the term parapsoriasis be retained any longer?

Since almost all patients with patch MF live a normal life, as do patients with parapsoriasis, whether one is a so called "lumper" or "splitter" should not matter; regardless of the name, patients generally follow a benign course. Although this is true, the diagnosis of MF places the patient in a cancer category, which had a negative impact on health and life insurance. Patients are not treated differently if one pathologist interprets their skin biopsy specimen as parapsoriasis and another as MF patch stage.

It is extremely rare for the author to receive a rule out diagnosis of parapsoriasis on a pathology requisition form. When parapsoriasis is in the differential diagnosis list, MF is invariably in the list as well. If the findings are those of early or patch MF, then it may be wise to report the diagnosis as MF, parapsoriasis type, just as dermatopathologists interpret lesions as squamous cell carcinoma, keratoacanthoma type.

The term parapsoriasis serves a historical purpose. Some dermatologists may choose to use it for patients with very limited and stable patches of MF in an attempt to avoid unnecessary anxiety about future health, mortality, and insurance.

Chapter 33
Red Sloughing Patches

Figure 33.1 illustrates two patients with two of the disorders discussed in this chapter.

Case A patient presents with diffusely red skin with pain and sloughing.
The clinical differential diagnosis includes

- acute phototoxicity,
- acute graft versus host disease,
- Paraneoplastic pemphigus,
- acute photosensitive lupus,
- staphylococcal scalded skin syndrome,
- Stevens Johnson syndrome SJS, and
- toxic epidermal necrolysis, TEN.

How Helpful Is the Pathology?

Only somewhat +/++

Clinical and Histological Differential Diagnosis

The clinical presentation of red, sloughing patches results from the process of "cytotoxic dermatitis" in which epidermal cells undergo death by apoptosis or other mechanisms. The histological findings are so similar that it is quite difficult to distinguish among the disorders based solely on histological findings. A biopsy from a patient with sloughing skin is valuable in excluding other disorders in which blistering occurs within the epidermis and without cell death, such as staph-scalded skin syndrome or extensive pemphigus.

The diagnosis of *acute phototoxicity* is usually easily made by the acute nature of the clinical presentation of a sunburn-like reaction in the presence of a phototoxic

D. F. Mutasim, *Practical Skin Pathology*, DOI 10.1007/978-3-319-14729-1_33

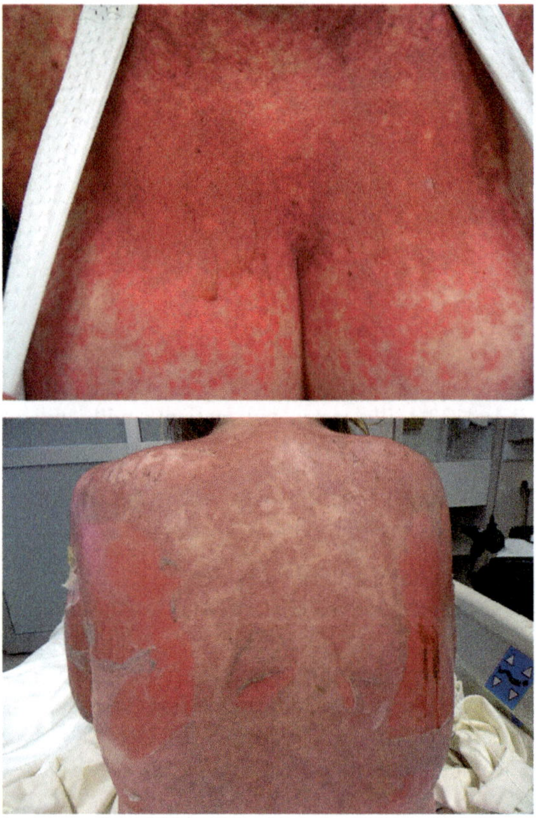

Fig. 33.1 *Upper panel* shows an elderly woman with painful deep erythema and focal sloughing caused by Stevens Johnson syndrome secondary to Dilantin received following brain surgery. *Lower panel* shows a middle-aged woman with deep redness and sloughing due to acute photoinduced lupus erythematosus as the initial presentation of systemic lupus erythematosus (SLE). Later, the patient developed extensive lesions of discoid lupus erythematosus and lupus panniculitis

medication. The histopathology is that of acute sunburn that is epidermal cell necrosis with no infiltrate. Later neutrophils may be seen in the epidermis.

The diagnosis of *acute graft versus host disease (GVHD)* is also generally easy to make in the right setting of recent bone marrow transplant. Grade 4 or severe acute GVHD results in full-thickness epidermal necrosis and sloughing.

The diagnosis of severe *acute photosensitive lupus* with epidermal necrosis is not as easy to make. This presentation of lupus is rare but may occur as the initial manifestation of systemic lupus erythematosus (SLE) when the patient is not yet known to have SLE with photosensitivity, and extremely rarely, subacute cutaneous lupus erythematosus (SCLE), in both disorders following extensive ultraviolet light exposure in an unsuspecting patient.

Unlike drug-induced phototoxicity, patients with acute photosensitive SLE may have oral erosions as well as evidence of vasculopathy of their fingers, toes, hands, and feet. Routine testing may reveal leukopenia, anemia, high sedimentation rate, proteinuria, and specific serologic tests for SLE antibodies help confirm the diagnosis.

The histology of lesions of acute photosensitive lupus, like that of the rare bullous lesions in SLE, is very different from the well-known findings of primary lesions of LE. While bullous lesions in SLE reveal a subepidermal vesicle with neutrophils, those in acute photosensitive lupus reveal epidermal necrosis and a minimal to no infiltrate, features that would not raise suspicion for lupus in the mind of the pathologist who is trained to suspect LE in the presence of a lymphocytic infiltrate. Instead, disorders such as toxic epidermal necrolysis (TEN) and Stevens–Johnson syndrome (SJS) are suspected.

So, how is a practitioner to confirm the diagnosis of SLE in a patient with diffusely sloughing skin, especially on sun-exposed areas? The answer is: by a high index of suspicion and ordering serological tests for SLE.

TEN and *SJS* are two closely related disorders with similar histopathology, identical etiology, and somewhat variable clinical presentation. The two disorders will be discussed together. Both present with extremely rapid pain, redness, and skin sloughing. Both reveal variable epidermal necrosis both in the form of individual keratinocytes and whole epidermis with usually minimal or no infiltrate and rarely a moderate infiltrate of lymphocytes that may contain eosinophils. Unlike TEN, some patients with SJS may have target lesions.

In infants and individuals with renal failure, the diagnosis of *staphylococcal scalded skin syndrome (SSSS)* is also considered in a patient with skin sloughing. Clues to the diagnosis of SSSS include a recent focus of *Staphylococcal* infection, lack of pain, and the character of the peeling tissue being stratum corneum not necrotic epidermis. A biopsy specimen is often diagnostic, whether processed for immediate frozen sections or permanent sections.

Paraneoplastic pemphigus may present clinically similarly to TEN. Indeed, many of the patients reported in the distant past as having TEN with pemphigus-like antibodies actually had PNP.

The diagnosis of *PNP* may be suspected *clinically* by:

1. A tendency towards a polymorphous eruption
2. Almost universal involvement of mucous membranes
3. More insidious onset than the other disorders in this category

PNP is as variable *histologically* as it is clinically. Only some cases have clearly evident suprabasilar acantholysis identical to pemphigus vulgaris (PV). Most cases reveal a variable combination of suprabasilar acantholysis like in pemphigus vulgaris and interface dermatitis like in erythema multiforme.

The diagnosis of PNP is made *immunologically* by:

1. Direct immunofluorescence. Compared to pemphigus vulgaris, PNP may have a lesser intensity of IgG and C3 deposition around epidermal cells, and frequently demonstrates C3 deposition along the basement membrane reminiscent of pemphigoid.
2. Indirect immunofluorescence reveals IgG antibodies not only against the cell surface of stratified squamous epithelium but also against simple and transitional epithelium, such as that of the gastrointestinal tract and urinary bladder, respectively.

So How Is the Diagnosis of PNP Confirmed? Most patients with PNP have an associated lymphoproliferative disorder that, in the majority of cases, is already known.

In patients suspected of having PNP, a search for an associated neoplasm is justified after attempting to confirm the diagnosis. This requires:

- Indirect immunofluorescence on special substrates including rat bladder. This test is only 80–85 % sensitive and specific for the diagnosis of PNP; hence, is not an absolute diagnostic criterion, whether positive or negative.
- Immunoprecipitation or ELISA performed on the patient's serum. This consistently reveals the characteristic set of antibodies that defines PNP, namely antibodies to desmogleins like in patients with PV and pemphigus foliaceous (PF), and additionally antibodies to desmosomal plaque proteins, which are not limited to stratified squamous epithelium. Neither of these tests is easily available.

What If the Diagnosis Is Still in Question Due to Unavailability of Special Tests or Nonspecific Results? The patient should undergo full evaluation for associated neoplasm particularly of the lymphoproliferative type (lymphocytic leukemia, B-cell lymphoma) usually with CT and/or PET-CT scans, examination of the peripheral blood, and possibly the bone marrow.

Conclusions

In the evaluation of a patient with red, tender sloughing skin, a combination of histological and ancillary studies is essential.

Chapter 34
Red Scaly Papules

Figure 34.1 illustrates two patients with two of the disorders discussed in this chapter.

Case A patient presents with acute eruption of multiple scaly, reddish papules over the trunk and extremities.

The *clinical differential diagnosis* on most pathology requisition forms for this presentation includes any number of the following four disorders:

- guttate psoriasis
- pityriasis rosea (PR)
- pityriasis lichenoides chronica (PLC), and
- secondary syphilis.

Clinical Clues

Unlike patients with the other disorders, patients with *PLC* report a chronic or waxing and waning eruption, and almost never present acutely. PLC is generally asymptomatic and follows a slow and insidious course; hence, patients present months after the onset of the first crop of lesions. Examination invariably reveals lesions at various stages of development and healing (red papules followed by finely scaly, thin flat-topped papules followed by brownish or hypo-pigmented macules).

Patients with secondary *syphilis* may present acutely with systemic symptoms, including low-grade fever and lymphadenopathy. They may or may not have evidence of primary chancre. They usually have mucosal and palmoplantar lesions.

Patients with papular *PR* also present acutely, reporting a rapidly progressive eruption. They may have a persistent or fading herald patch. Even when the lesions are papules (which occurs more frequently in dark-skinned individuals), the eruption still respects the so-called Christmas-tree pattern and upon close inspection, some papules may show a collarette of fine scale.

D. F. Mutasim, *Practical Skin Pathology*, DOI 10.1007/978-3-319-14729-1_34

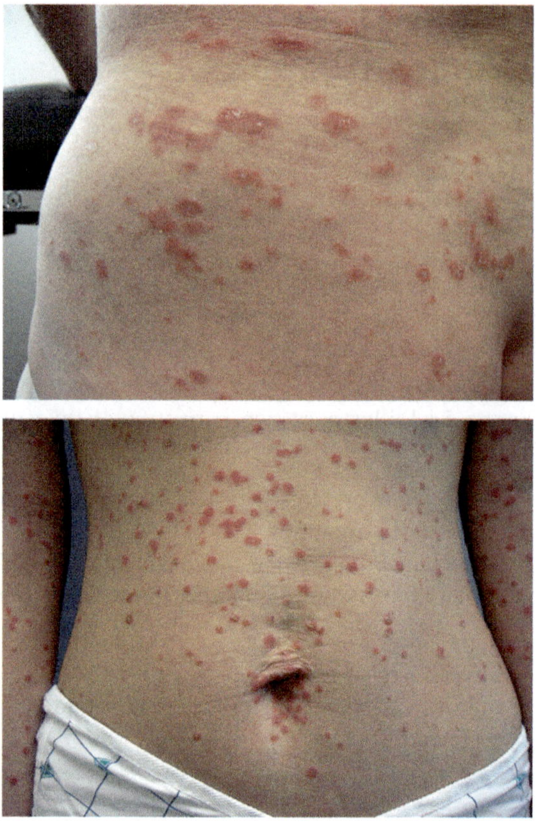

Fig. 34.1 *Upper panel* reveals a middle-aged woman who presented with a 2-week history of an asymptomatic papulosquamous eruption characteristic of pityriasis rosea. *Lower panel* reveals a young woman with eruptive guttate psoriasis

Finally, most patients with the first episode of acute *guttate psoriasis* recall a recent upper respiratory infection. Guttate psoriasis lesions tend to be more intensely red than papules of PR, PLC, and secondary syphilis.

A *drug eruption* may occasionally be papulosquamous, especially mimicking PR.

How Helpful Is the Pathology?

Very helpful +++

In the above clinical presentation, two or more biopsies should result in an accurate diagnosis in practically all cases. The need for more than one biopsy is due to the fact that the diagnostic findings of guttate psoriasis and PLC are present in a short phase in the evolutionary life of each lesion. The histological findings in the two disorders are so dynamic that a very early or very old lesion may miss the diagnostic findings.

Histological Findings

The earliest lesion of *guttate psoriasis* may reveal spongiosis and only minimal focal parakeratosis with only slight focal atrophy of the granular layer beneath foci of parakeratosis. The tortuous capillaries characteristic of mature or plaque psoriasis have not formed yet. Hence, differentiation from spongiotic dermatitis and PR may be difficult.

A several-day-old lesion of guttate psoriasis would likely reveal parakeratosis, neutrophils in the horny layer, less spongiosis, and the beginning of epidermal hyperplasia that is not regular yet. A mild superficial perivascular infiltrate does not add or take support away from the diagnosis. This combination of the above findings in the appropriate clinical setting should confirm the diagnosis of guttate psoriasis against PR and PLC. If plasma cells and/or histiocytes are abundant, then secondary syphilis should be strongly considered.

Similarly, during the 2-to-3-week total life of a lesion of *PLC*, it goes through so many changes that the histological findings also vary depending on the age of the lesion. In the "mature" pinkish, finely scaled, flat-topped, thin papule of PLC, the textbook findings are easily identified. These consist of a plate of parakeratosis, only mild acanthosis, mild–to-moderate basal vacuolization and a generally mild interface, and superficial perivascular lymphocytic infiltrate with no other cell type. The lack of neutrophils in the horny layer and the presence of an intact granular layer, as well as basal vacuolization, all help support the diagnosis of PLC over guttate psoriasis. The lack of spongiosis and the presence of basal vacuolization speak against the diagnosis of PR.

Lesions of *PR* are also dynamic, but to a lesser degree than guttate psoriasis and PLC. The histological findings of PR are those of subacute spongiotic dermatitis. Features that may favor PR over other causes of subacute spongiotic dermatitis include parakeratosis in the form of mounds, extravasation of red cells, and occasional mild dyskeratosis. These clues may be missing or so mild that unless PR is being clinically suspected on the requisition form, the diagnosis may not be considered by the pathologist; hence, the importance of providing clinical findings and differential diagnosis to the pathologist.

In the case of generally asymptomatic scaly patches and thin papules of recent onset, a histological diagnosis of subacute spongiotic dermatitis should be taken by the clinician as highly supportive of PR.

In *secondary syphilis*, there is no single histological finding that is diagnostic. Just as the clinical lesions in secondary syphilis are polymorphous (macules, papules, plaques, and nodules), so are the histological findings. In addition, the age of the eruption, which may last up to a year dictates to a large extent the histological findings as older lesions are more likely to become granulomatous and reveal abundant histiocytes, sometimes forming granulomas.

Lesions of secondary syphilis may have the findings of *psoriasiform* dermatitis, *lichenoid* dermatitis, *granulomatous* dermatitis, or combination of two or three. As for the composition of the infiltrate, in addition to some lymphocytes, plasma cells and or histiocytes are very helpful in suspecting the diagnosis. Unlike guttate psoriasis, PR, and PLC, the infiltrate in secondary syphilis involves the deeper dermal plexus in addition to the superficial plexus. The following are histological presentations that should strongly raise suspicion for secondary syphilis:

1. A *psoriasiform* dermatitis that does not conform to psoriasis, PRP, or lichenified dermatitis, and that has a deeper infiltrate, and/or histiocytes, and/or plasma cells is almost certainly secondary syphilis.
2. A *lichenoid* interface dermatitis that does not conform to the diagnosis of lichen planus, and that also reveals some degree of psoriasiform epidermal hyperplasia, a deeper component to the infiltrate, with histiocytes, and/or plasma cells, and absence of epidermotropism is almost certainly secondary syphilis.
3. A *histiocytic*/granulomatous infiltrate that does not conform to sarcoidosis and related disorders and that extends to the deep dermis, and that contains abundant plasma cells, and arranged haphazardly around blood vessels and in the interstitial spaces rather than in well-defined granulomas is almost certainly secondary syphilis.

Finally patients with secondary syphilis have positive syphilis serology 100% of the time.

Conclusions

In the evaluation of patients with an acute eruption of red, scaly papules, more than one biopsy specimen is often needed to make an accurate diagnosis.

Chapter 35
Red Non-Facial Papules

Figure 35.1 illustrates two patients with two of the disorders discussed in this chapter.

Case A patient presents with itchy, red papules scattered over the trunk and/or extremities. Some or many lesions may be excoriated. Only a rare lesion may be lichenified, appearing as prurigo nodularis. New lesions appear at variable intervals, and each lesion may last for a few days to few weeks.

The quality of life of most patients who present as above is compromised and many have been to allergists and/or a few dermatologists expecting an answer as to the cause of the lesions and/or a cure. Some may have diagnosed themselves as allergic to something or another, and others have declared themselves or were told to be gluten-sensitive. Most of them are resistant to topical steroids including super-potent ones. Most patients respond dramatically to systemic steroids.

The *differential diagnosis* of the above presentation includes:

A. Disorders with identifiable etiology such as:

- Insect bite reaction, including mites and pediculosis
- Scabies
- Drug eruption
- "Neutrophilic dermatosis" secondary to any of multiple systemic disorders, and

B. Disorders without identifiable etiology, namely, the idiopathic disorder(s) that has been named at different times, in different countries, and by different authors as prurigo simplex, subacute prurigo, prurigo mitis, "itchy red bump disease", and hypersensitivity reaction.

In the evaluation of these patients, two groups of disorders should be excluded, namely:

- Patients with generalized pruritus and excoriations without primary lesions (discussed in Chap. 27)
- Patients with delusions of parasitosis and secondary excoriations, without primary lesions

D. F. Mutasim, *Practical Skin Pathology*, DOI 10.1007/978-3-319-14729-1_35

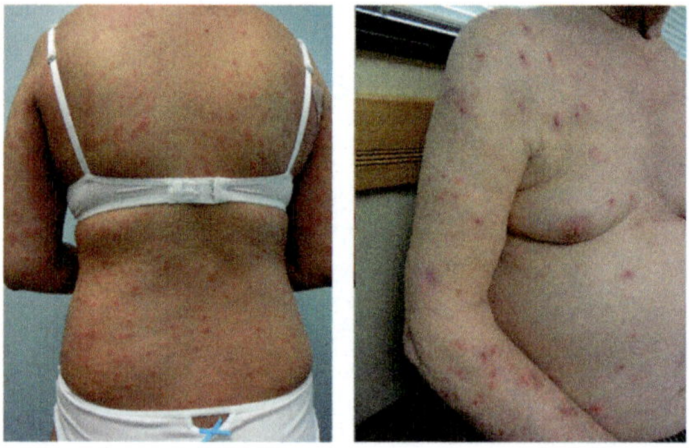

Fig. 35.1 *Left panel* demonstrates a pregnant woman with generalized eruption of red papules characteristic of pruritic urticarial papules and plaques of pregnancy. *Right panel* demonstrates an old man with idiopathic, severely pruritic papules that he excoriates. Histological examination of a rare primary lesion revealed the findings of hypersensitivity reaction or prurigo simplex

Clinical Clues

Patients with scabies almost always have genital lesions, especially in males. Another clue may be the extreme severity of the itching. Scabies may be by far the most pruritic disorder in dermatology. Patients wake up at night due to itching.

Bite reactions vary in symptoms and morphology (papules, hives, nodules, bullae, and combinations). History is often helpful.

The remaining disorders in this group have many overlapping features, and cannot be distinguished based solely on clinical examination.

How Helpful Is the Pathology?

Moderately ++

Two distinct histological patterns characterize the lesions in this section. First, a lymphocytic and eosinophilic infiltrate; and second, a neutrophil-rich infiltrate.

Lymphocytic and Eosinophilic

In the first and much more common histological presentation, biopsies of red papules reveal a variable perivascular infiltrate of lymphocytes and eosinophils. The number of eosinophils varies from only a few to many. Histological identification of a cause is most often not possible.

If the overlying epidermis is also involved in the inflammatory process, that is, there is spongiosis and exocytosis with or without parakeratosis and acanthosis, then the finding most likely represents an *insect bite reaction* or *scabies*. Unless a component of the scabies mite is detected, the histological diagnosis can only be "insect bite reaction or scabies." It is important here to remember that the vast majority of papules in patients with scabies are secondary to the development of immune response to the mite products rather than to direct infestation by scabies organisms.

If the overlying epidermis is unremarkable or reveals only an excoriation, then the differential diagnosis is much wider and would include, in addition to insect bite reaction and scabies, the *idiopathic* disorder that carries many names (prurigo simplex, subacute prurigo, prurigo mitis, "itchy red bump disease," and hypersensitivity reaction).

How about *drug reaction*? Is there a histological finding that would confirm or at least suggest the etiology as medication? The answer is "no." Some consider the presence of eosinophils to strongly suggest drug etiology, whether the infiltrate is that of hypersensitivity reaction (discussed extensively elsewhere), lichen planus, or leukocytoclastic vasculitis.

How about *urticaria*? In the absence of epidermal involvement, a perivascular and interstitial infiltrate of lymphocytes and eosinophils is characteristic of urticaria. The clinical lesions, however, are transient hives rather than papules and are easily distinguishable.

How about a *paraneoplastic* disorder? Rarely, itchy red papules mimicking lesions of insect bite reaction are a manifestation of an acquired immune deficiency or hematological malignancy such as leukemia. These patients have lesions that appear characteristic of insect bite reaction yet with convincing lack of evidence for exposure to insects. Patients with this presentation usually are known to have the diagnosis of immune deficiency or hematological malignancy.

Neutrophilic

In this less frequent histological presentation, there is a perivascular and often interstitial infiltrate of neutrophils that tends to be mild to moderate, with or without dermal edema. There is no vasculitis or significant papillary dermal edema; so LCV and Sweet syndrome are easily excluded.

This histological finding is usually reported as "neutrophilic dermatosis" or something close, such as "consistent with neutrophilic urticaria" or "suggestive of urticarial vasculitis," two disorders in which the lesions are transient and urticarial rather than persistent papules.

Patients with this histological picture are often known to have a systemic disorder such as rheumatoid arthritis, SLE, inflammatory bowel disease, intestinal bypass surgery, and the like. If not known, then evaluation is required. This dermatological presentation rarely goes without an associated systemic disorder; hence, continued search for one is indicated if the initial evaluation is negative.

Rarely, red papules that wax and wane in a child may represent chronic meningococcal infection. Lesions tend to be short-lived, and a biopsy may be delayed. The diagnosis usually requires a high index of suspicion, especially in the presence of fever. In the proper setting, a neutrophilic infiltrate with or without vasculitis is highly consistent with the diagnosis of chronic meningococcal infection.

Conclusions

In the evaluation of patients with multiple itchy, red papules, histopathology is of moderate value.

Chapter 36
Papulonodular Lesions with Scale and/or Crust

Figure 36.1 illustrates two patients with two of the disorders discussed in this chapter.

Case A patient presents with a several month history of multiple scattered papules and nodules, some crusted.

Clinical differential diagnosis includes

- pityriasis lichenoides et varioliformis acuta PLEVA
- lymphomatoid papulosis LyP
- secondary syphilis
- nodular scabies
- prurigo nodularis PN
- nodular pemphigoid NP and
- disseminated infection.

Clinical Clues

Children with the above presentation are more likely to have PLEVA, bites, or scabies. NP favors the elderly. Disseminated infection often occurs in immunosuppressed individuals.

Lesions that vary in morphology with time and some of which heal with scar strongly favor PLEVA and LyP (classic type), while lesions that are pruritic and appear lichenified are likely PN more often than nodular scabies and NP. Genital lesions favor scabies; mucosal lesions favor secondary syphilis.

How Helpful Is the Pathology?

Very helpful+++

There is almost no overlap among the histological features between the above seven disorders.

D. F. Mutasim, *Practical Skin Pathology*, DOI 10.1007/978-3-319-14729-1_36

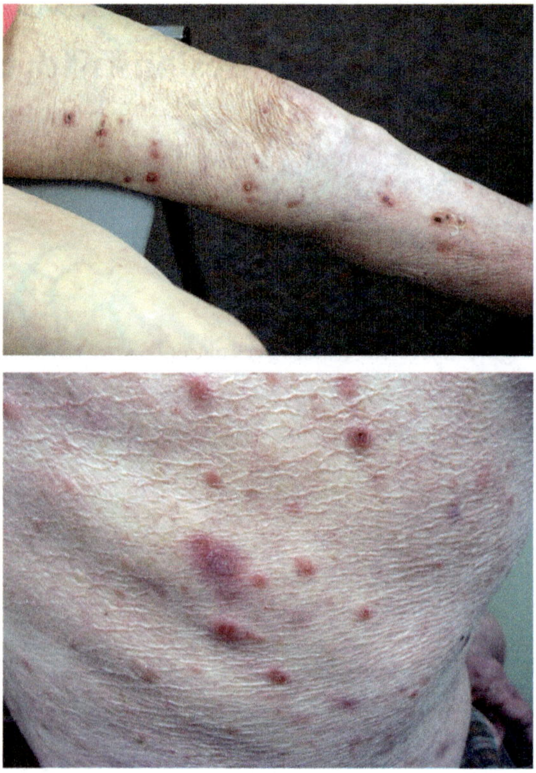

Fig. 36.1 *Upper panel* reveals an older woman with disseminated dermal papules and pustules over one leg secondary to atypical mycobacterial infection. *Lower panel* reveals an old man with severe lymphomatoid papulosis. The patient also had mycosis fungoides and limited primary cutaneous CD30 positive lymphoma

Histological Findings

A mature lesion of *PLEVA* that is a red papule with a surface change of both scale and mild crust before the phase of the erosion, and after the phase of smooth, red papule shows such characteristic changes that the diagnosis may be made with absolute certainty. The findings include diffuse parakeratosis, loss of the granular layer replaced by pale superficial epidermis, regular acanthosis, moderate dyskeratosis, basal vacuolization, and a generally moderate, purely lymphocytic infiltrate in the superficial and (to a lesser degree) the deep dermis. The monomorphous nature of the infiltrate is quite characteristic. The presence of other cell types denies the diagnosis of PLEVA. Extravasated red cells may be seen both in the papillary dermis as well as in the epidermis.

In the characteristic intermediate-age lesion of classic *LyP*, the epidermal findings may or may not mimic those in PLEVA, but the diagnostic findings are those in the dermis. In the classical nodular presentation of LyP described in the original paper, the dermal infiltrate is most often that of so-called histological type A LyP, that is, a moderate-to-dense, superficial and deep mixed infiltrate of small lymphocytes, scattered, large lymphocytes, and other inflammatory cell types that may include neutrophils and histiocytes as well as eosinophils. In some cases, eosinophils may be abundant, raising suspicion sometimes for a reaction to insect bite.

The so-called type B LyP is characterized clinically by small papules (often referred to as papular LyP) and reveals findings similar to those in mycosis fungoides (MF) and may be distinguished only by the clinical presentation and the tendency of lesions of LyP to spontaneously involute.

PN, NP, nodular scabies, and nodular syphilis all share significant epidermal hyperplasia but differ in ways that makes differentiation among the four disorders rather easy.

In lesions of *PN* there is hyperkeratosis, often severe epidermal hyperplasia, papillary dermal fibrosis, and a highly variable superficial infiltrate that varies from "minimal or nonexistent" all the way to intense, with lymphocytes and sometimes numerous eosinophils.

Lesions of *NP* share similar features to PN. In order to suspect what was first thought to be PN may indeed be NP requires the presence of:

- Eosinophils not only in the papillary dermal infiltrate but also along the dermal epidermal junction
- Eosinophil exocytosis, especially in association with spongiosis, the so-called eosinophilic spongiosis
- Small cleft(s) in the dermal–epidermal junction

Nodular scabies is a diagnosis based mostly on dermal findings. The epidermis may be unremarkable, spongiotic, and/or hyperplastic. Mites are seldom found in the horny layer within a lesion of nodular scabies. The characteristic dermal findings are those of a "persistent hypersensitivity reaction" or "pseudolymphoma". Both, the superficial and deep dermis, are invariably involved with a usually dense infiltrate of lymphocytes with many eosinophils. The infiltrate is primarily perivascular but may be focally nodular and/or diffuse raising suspicion for lymphoma. The differential diagnosis of nodular scabies histologically is persistent insect bite reaction, from which it is differentiated by clinical examination.

Nodular syphilis may share epidermal hyperplasia with the above three disorders but differs significantly in the composition of the infiltrate which, in addition to lymphocytes, very frequently contains plasma cells and/or histiocytes, and lacks eosinophils. Patients with nodular syphilis have positive syphilis serology.

Conclusions

In the setting of a papular/nodular eruption, the clinical and histological findings should lead to an accurate diagnosis all the time.

Chapter 37
Edematous Smooth Plaques

Figure 37.1 illustrates two patients with two of the disorders discussed in this chapter.

Case A patient presents with a recent onset of a diffuse eruption of reddish, edematous, smooth plaques without scaling or crusting; an occasional lesion may be annular.

Clinical differential diagnosis includes

- urticaria (acute or chronic)
- urticarial vasculitis UV
- urticarial pemphigoid
- Sweet syndrome
- neutrophilic eccrine hidradenitis NEH
- erythema multiforme EM
- fixed drug eruption FDE
- tumid lupus erythematosus TLE, and
- polymorphous light eruption PMLE.

Clinical Clues

Lesions of *urticaria*, whether acute or chronic, resolve within few hours, leaving behind no discoloration or other traces. Lesions are usually pruritic.

In contradistinction, lesions of *UV*, usually last longer than 24 h and up to a few days. Upon resolution, discoloration is almost invariable and may appear slightly purplish, purpuric, or brownish. Lesions of UV produce a burning rather than itchy sensation.

The prodromal pre-blistering eruption of *pemphigoid* is characteristically urticarial. Unlike lesions of urticaria, the non-bullous lesions of pemphigoid are more infiltrated and persist for days to weeks, if not treated. Not infrequently, very close inspection may reveal one or more minute, clear vesicles within the urticarial

D. F. Mutasim, *Practical Skin Pathology*, DOI 10.1007/978-3-319-14729-1_37

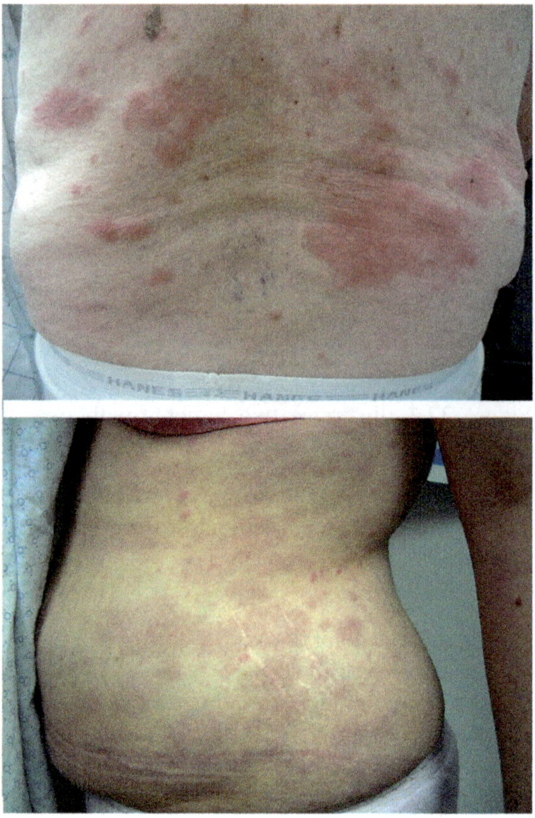

Fig. 37.1 *Upper panel* demonstrates an older man with smooth edematous plaques of urticarial pemphigoid. *Lower panel* demonstrates a woman with smooth edematous plaques of urticarial vasculitis

plaque, including at the border. The distribution of lesions of urticarial pemphigoid may not respect the usual distribution of lesions in patients with bullous pemphigoid, which favors skin folds.

Lesions of *Sweet syndrome* are often fiery red, burning and painful, may be tender, often boggy, and persistent. Their classic acral distribution is a good clue to the diagnosis. In the full syndrome, also referred to as classic Sweet syndrome, fever and leukocytosis are major clues.

An eruption of red edematous plaques may rarely be caused by *neutrophilic eccrine hidradenitis*. Many patients would be known to have an associated systemic illness or be on systemic chemotherapy. Lesions may favor the skin of the palms and soles.

EM is almost invariably symmetrical and the majority of patients have at least some target lesions. *FDE* lesions tend to be few, larger than lesions of EM and scattered asymmetrically. They often favor mucocutaneous junctions of the mouth and genitalia, and are often pigmented.

TLE and *PMLE* may appear similar clinically, both as soft smooth papules and nodules or plaques. Lesions of TLE, however, may be scattered anywhere on the skin surface, including the face and neck; while the eruption of PMLE is usually symmetrical, strongly favors the extremities, and rarely involves the face.

How Helpful Is the Pathology?

Very helpful+++

Histological Findings

Both, *urticaria* and *urticarial vasculitis* have infiltrates that surround dermal blood vessels. In urticaria, there is an infiltrate of lymphocytes and a variable number of eosinophils with or without few neutrophils. In urticarial vasculitis, the infiltrate is almost exclusively neutrophils with or without a few eosinophils, sometimes with nuclear dust, red blood cells, and extension of the neutrophils into blood vessel walls with usually mild fibrin deposition. Hence, the differentiation between the two disorders should be straightforward. Occasionally, however, the findings are intermediate, that is, the findings are those of urticaria, but in addition to eosinophils there is abundance or predominance of neutrophils without vessel wall involvement. Most pathologists refer to this histological picture as "*neutrophilic urticaria.*"

Neutrophilic urticaria lesions may be intermediate in symptomatology between urticaria and urticarial vasculitis in that patients may volunteer the symptom of burning. The exact nosology of neutrophilic urticaria is, however, not clear. I have seen a rare patient in whom some lesions revealed the histological findings of neutrophilic urticaria; while others revealed the findings of urticarial vasculitis. Therefore, if the clinical suspicion for urticarial vasculitis is high, and only one biopsy is obtained and reported as "neutrophilic urticarial," further biopsies would be indicated to look for the possibility of urticarial vasculitis. In such instances, direct immunofluorescence may be helpful if it reveals prominent immune complex deposition in dermal blood vessel walls.

The diagnosis of *urticarial pemphigoid* should be strongly suspected in a biopsy specimen of a fixed urticarial lesion if the infiltrate is limited to the papillary dermis, and contains eosinophils, some of which tagging the demo–epidermal junction. The presence of eosinophilic exocytosis and spongiosis (eosinophilic spongiosis) is further support for the diagnosis of pemphigoid (whether classical or pregnancy associated).

The histological findings of *Sweet syndrome* are so classical that the diagnosis is easily made at the scanning magnification of a lesion that reveals papillary dermal edema and a diffuse infiltrate of neutrophils with minimal or no nuclear dust in the superficial dermis. The diffuse nature of the infiltrate and the lack of vasculitis exclude vasculitis and other types of neutrophilic dermatosis. Combined with the clinical findings, the diagnosis of Sweet syndrome is often made with a high degree of certainty.

NEH is one of few disorders in which the clinical findings are far more impressive than the histological findings. On scanning magnification, sections reveal almost normal skin. Only on closer inspection or deeper sectioning may the characteristic neutrophilic infiltrate surrounding the eccrine glands in the deep dermis or subcutaneous fat reveal itself. Rarely does the infiltrate of NEH go beyond the eccrine coils.

Therefore, if a biopsy specimen is small or superficial, and deeper sections are not obtained, the findings might be so sparse that the diagnosis may be missed. In the face of red edematous plaques with minimal histology, the diagnosis of NEH should be strongly suspected.

EM is a predominantly acral eruption just as Sweet syndrome. Most patients with EM have target lesions and many patients with recurrent EM provide history for recurrent HSV infection. Dyskeratosis is a reliable finding although variable in degree. Basal cell vacuolization is also a reliable finding, along with superficial lymphocytic infiltrate. A few melanophages may be present.

The histological diagnosis of *FDE* is generally very easy, at least in the second episode and afterwards, when the hyperpigmentation is evident. During the first episode, however, clinical clues to the diagnosis include involvement of mucocutaneous junction of the oral and genital area. Lesions are characteristically round and generally few in numbers. In clinically atypical presentations, the diagnosis may be made histologically and differentiated from EM by generally more severe dyskeratosis that may progress into complete epidermal necrosis and blistering or sloughing-off, the presence of many superficial melanophages, and a tendency for the infiltrate to extend deeper than the papillary dermis and be polymorphous, that is, containing few neutrophils and eosinophils.

Lesions of *TLE* may be plaques, papules, and or nodules. The epidermis is usually unremarkable or reveals mild and sometimes overlooked vacuolization of basal cells. The superficial and deep reticular dermis reveal a mild to moderate lymphocytic infiltrate and mucin is almost invariably present.

Lesions of *PMLE* also have a dermal lymphocytic infiltrate but without mucin. Frequently, there is marked papillary dermal edema with extravasated red cells.

Conclusions

At least one and preferably two full-thickness skin biopsies should lead to an accurate diagnosis in a patient presenting with multiple reddish, edematous, smooth plaques in almost 100 % of cases. Since most of the above disorders are manifestations of hypersensitivity to a medication or systemic illness, making the clinical diagnosis is only a prelude to searching for its cause.

Chapter 38
Sclerotic Plaques

Figure 38.1 illustrates two patients with two of the disorders discussed in this chapter.

Case A person presents with discrete sclerotic smooth plaques.

Clinical differential diagnosis includes

- morphea (the most common diagnosis)
- lichen sclerosis (LS)
- some cases of early atrophoderma
- chronic radiation dermatitis
- scleromyxedema, and
- nephrogenic systemic fibrosis (NSF).

Scleroderma, whether diffuse or limited, is excluded due to the discrete nature of the eruption. Scleredema, although not a truly sclerotic disorder but dermal thickening may appear grossly sclerotic; however, patients are diffusely affected.

Clinical Clues

Common Disorders

Clinical clues here are extremely helpful. The clinical characteristics of plaque lesions of *morphea* whether localized or generalized are well known to the dermatology practitioners. A whitish surface that is rough to the touch due to hyperkeratosis is characteristic of *lichen sclerosis*, and a brownish hue with cliff border is characteristic of *atrophoderma*.

The end-stage of morphea and the (older) center of old lesions may acquire an ivory color reminiscent of the white color of lichen sclerosis so that the two disorders may be occasionally confused. This is especially true when the two disorders

D. F. Mutasim, *Practical Skin Pathology*, DOI 10.1007/978-3-319-14729-1_38

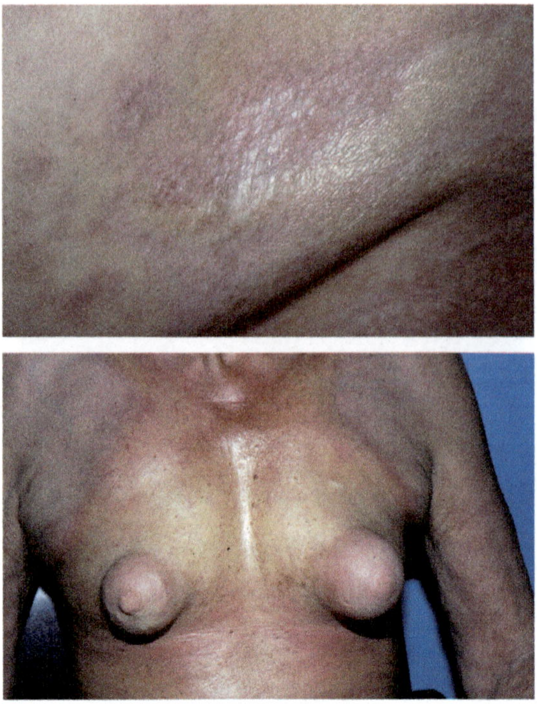

Fig. 38.1 *Upper panel* shows an elderly woman with lesions that had the clinical and histological findings of both morphea and lichen sclerosis. *Lower panel* shows an elderly woman who presented with severe limitation to breathing and shrinkage of her breast tissue due to encasement of her chest by tight firm skin of morphea profunda

coexist in the same patient or the same lesion. In general, the induration in morphea (due to sclerosis in the whole reticular dermis) is much thicker and deeper than that in LS (in which sclerosis is limited to the papillary dermis).

The relationship between atrophoderma and morphea has been debated since the initial descriptions of atrophoderma, decades ago. Some authors propose that atrophoderma is a type of morphea, while others consider it a unique disorder.

Those in favor of atrophoderma being a type of morphea refer to the observation that an involuted or healed lesion of morphea may appear similar to lesions of atrophoderma, and that an early or active lesion of atrophoderma reveals similar, although milder, histological findings to morphea, namely, sclerosis and lymphocytic infiltrate. In addition, there are several reports of patients having a combination of lesions, some characteristic of morphea and others characteristic of atrophoderma, clinically and histologically. I have seen few such patients. I have also seen patients who have classic lesions of atrophoderma and who, years later, develop lesions clinically and histologically characteristic of plaque morphea.

On the other hand, those against the idea that atrophoderma is a type of morphea emphasize the observation that most patients who have findings similar to what is termed atrophoderma never report history of or provide documentation of lesions with features of morphea clinically or histologically and that, unlike morphea, many patients with atrophoderma have a solitary large lesion of the trunk with characteristic borders very early in its course.

The debate may continue as long as the etiology of both disorders is unknown. Whether atrophoderma is viewed as a type of morphea or not, the clinical and histological characteristics are unique enough to justify using the term atrophoderma as the primary diagnosis. To diagnose it as morphea clinically or histologically does not serve to advance the understanding of its nosology.

Similar arguments have been made as to the nature of LS. Some argue that it is a subtype of morphea, namely, a superficial type involving the papillary dermis. In support of this view is the observation that the disorder is characterized by papillary dermal sclerosis. The fact that morphea and lichen sclerosis may coexist in the same lesion or the same patient has also been used in support of this view.

Others, including the author, favor the view that LS is unique. The fact that LS frequently involves and may be limited to the anogenital area, which is not known to be involved by morphea, and the fact that genital lesions are precancerous make LS a unique disorder. Again, there is no benefit to our understanding of either disorder to lump LS under morphea.

Uncommon Disorders

Both, chronic radiation dermatitis and scleromyxedema appear sclerotic upon palpation. The other findings of *chronic radiation dermatitis*, however, are so characteristic (irregular telangiectasias, variable hyperkeratosis, purpura, and pallor) that the clinical diagnosis is rarely missed. Plaques of *scleromyxedema* and the closely related disorder, *NSF*, usually having a brownish hue are raised and are sometimes associated with papules.

How Helpful Is the Pathology?

Very helpful+++

Histological Clues

The histological findings of *morphea* (reticular dermal sclerosis associated with a superficial and deep perivascular and interstitial lymphocytes with or without plasma cells) can hardly be missed even at scanning magnification. Similarly, the characteristic findings of *LS* (papillary dermal edema followed by sclerosis and a perivascular often band-like infiltrate at the junction between the papillary dermis and the uninvolved reticular dermis) are also hardly missed.

The histological findings of *atrophoderma*, on the other hand, can be easily missed. Along with ichthyosis, tinea versicolor, hyper- and hypopigmentary disorders, and other disorders with subtle histological findings, the histological diagnosis of atrophoderma may easily be missed. Although a mild infiltrate may be seen in the very early lesions, by the time patients present to the dermatologist, the infiltrate has disappeared and the only evidence of pathology left is a decreased thickness of the reticular dermis without obvious sclerosis.

Without being alerted by the clinician that atrophoderma is a possible diagnosis, a pathologist will likely miss the diagnosis. A pathologist would only make the diagnosis if the biopsy specimen is a long, incisional biopsy that includes involved skin, the border, and adjacent normal skin. Alternatively, a biopsy from the center of the lesion and another from normal skin in the immediate vicinity of the lesion would be helpful as long as they include fat. This way, the thickness of the dermis can be measured and determined to be decreased in the lesion compared to normal adjacent skin.

Chronic radiation dermatitis is striking in the variability of findings in the same specimen. The thickness of the horny layer and that of the epidermis vary so that there may be acanthosis adjacent to atrophy. The basal cells may appear atypical, disorganized, and squamatized. The dermis is generally hyalinized, may be focally degenerated, and edematous with paucity of adnexal structures. Blood vessels are irregularly dilated, and many may be filled with red cells. The stroma is often purpuric. In long-standing lesions, the epidermis may reveal changes of radiation keratosis or squamous cell carcinoma. The appearance of collagen is too distinctive to be missed for lichen sclerosis, the disorder that is often taught in the differential diagnosis.

Finally, *scleromyxedema* and *NSF* reveal proliferation of fibroblasts and excessive interstitial mucin in addition to collagen thickening. In a small biopsy, differentiation from papular mucinosis/lichen myxedematosis may be difficult.

Conclusions

Except in atrophoderma, one biopsy of full-thickness skin leads to a specific diagnosis in patients with sclerotic plaques almost always. For differentiation between scleromyxedema and NSF, history is essential.

Chapter 39
Diffuse Sclerosis

Figure 39.1 illustrates two patients with two of the disorders discussed in this chapter.

Case A patient presents with diffuse thickening of the skin involving a large area of their skin.

Clinical differential diagnosis includes

- scleroderma (both diffuse and limited)
- chronic graft versus host disease (GVHD)
- eosinophilic fasciitis (EF)
- scleredema, and less likely
- nephrogenic systemic fibrosis (NSF), and
- scleromyxedema.

The latter two disorders more often present with discrete lesions. Similarly, generalized morphea consists of discrete lesions and can be differentiated easily.

Clinical Clues

Patients with *scleroderma*, whether diffuse or limited, usually have acral sclerosis and sclerodactyly as well as history of Raynaud's phenomenon. Other manifestations may include fingertip infarcts, telangiectasias, salt and pepper pigmentation especially over the upper back, and calcinosis. Some patients may have internal organ involvement, particularly the lungs and kidneys. Patients with generalized morphea should not be confused with scleroderma.

The primary manifestation of *chronic GVHD* is sclerodermoid skin changes akin to those of scleroderma. Without history of a bone marrow transplant, the two disorders may be difficult to differentiate. Features that may favor chronic GVHD include residual findings of subacute and rarely acute GVHD, that is, lichenoid papules and erythema. History of acute GVHD is almost universally elicited.

D. F. Mutasim, *Practical Skin Pathology*, DOI 10.1007/978-3-319-14729-1_39

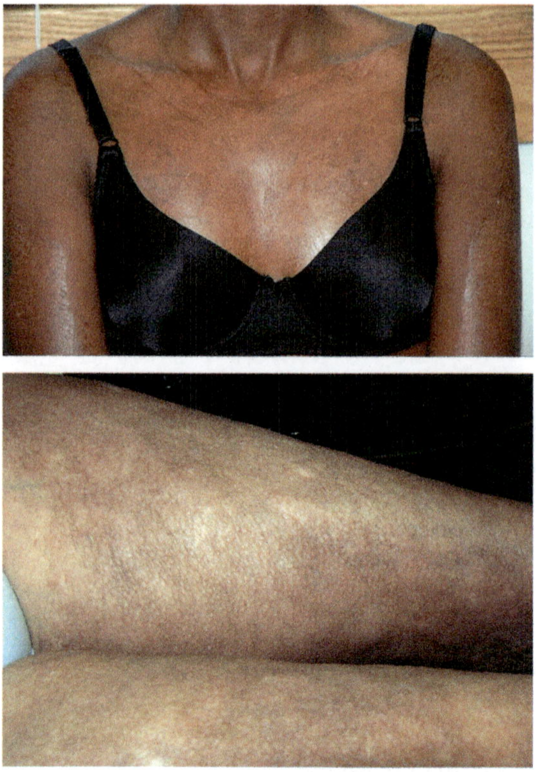

Fig. 39.1 *Upper panel* reveals a young woman with diffuse scleroderma, loss of multiple fingers, and severe pulmonary disease. *Lower panel* reveals a middle-aged woman with renal failure and nephrogenic systemic fibrosis. The brownish skin of her thighs was deeply indurated

Patients with *EF* present either as acute–onset, painful, rapid induration of the skin of the extremities, especially the legs (reported in male runners in the initial report by Dr. Shulman), or as insidious progressive thickening of the skin diffusely, commonly with overlying *peau de orange* appearance of the skin surface that may be difficult to distinguish from subcutaneous morphea, also known as morphea profunda.

In my experience, the two disorders may be closely related and are not always easy to differentiate from each other; hence, explaining the multiple histological diagnoses given to patients with such a presentation. I have seen patients who have brought pathology reports, some of which interpreted as morphea profunda and others as EF. This difference in interpretation may be partly due to pathologists' personal understanding of the two disease processes but often is due to the difference in the available tissue submitted for histological evaluation.

Patients with EF are well known to have sclerosis extending outward into the overlying dermis, leading to interpreting a superficial biopsy specimen from such patients as morphea. The course and response to treatment of both EF and morphea profunda are so similar that for practical clinical purposes, the two disorders may be viewed as closely related points on the spectrum of cutaneous and subcutaneous sclerosis.

Patients with *scleromyxedema* and *NSF* share many features, both clinically and histologically, that in the absence of history of renal failure and exposure to gadolinium in MRI study, the two disorders may not be differentiated with absolute certainty in all cases.

Patients with *scleredema* present with thickening of the skin without any surface changes, such as discoloration or peau de orange appearance. Patients usually have limitation of motion of the neck and shoulders. A predisposing factor that may be elicited is diabetes in adults and streptococcal infection in children.

How Helpful Is the Pathology?

Only moderately +/++

Histological Clues

Both morphea and scleroderma demonstrate sclerotic collagen throughout the dermis. Compared to *morphea*, which often reveals at least mild and often moderate lymphocytic infiltrate with possible plasma cells in both the superficial and deep vascular plexus, lesions of *scleroderma* lack a similar infiltrate; hence, the two disorders are often possible to differentiate histologically.

The findings in *chronic GVHD* are similar to those in scleroderma. In addition, interface changes of subacute GVHD may be present. These may be epidermal hyperplasia, basal vacuolization, and melanophages. In some cases, findings reminiscent of lichen planus are evident.

As mentioned above, differentiation between *EF* and *morphea profunda* may be extremely difficult. If the specimen extends only to the deep reticular dermis then only a diagnosis of morphea may be made. For the diagnosis of EF to be confirmed an incisional biopsy specimen containing subcutaneous fat and underlying fascia is required. Even then pathologists may differ in their interpretation of sclerosis extending from the dermis through the subcutaneous fat into the fascia. It is difficult to determine whether the primary site of pathology is in the fascia which then is extended outward, or whether it is in the reticular dermis and extended inward. The presence of eosinophils, although helpful, is not diagnostic of EF. An excellent study has shown that tissue and circulating eosinophilia may be seen in morphea and scleroderma, albeit in a lesser frequency and number than EF.

In the face of similar course and response (or lack thereof) to treatment in both disorders, differentiating between the two disorders may be academic.

Thickening of the skin in *scleredema* results from excessive deposition of (non-sclerotic) collagen and ground substance, that is mucin. Some cases have only small amount of mucin. The diagnosis in these cases may be missed if the biopsy is superficial. The thickness of the dermis in scleredema measures two to three times that of normal skin at the site of involvement.

Conclusions

Thorough clinical evaluation of the patient with diffuse thickening of the skin is often more helpful than histopathology.

Chapter 40
Purpuric Lesions

Figure 40.1 illustrates two patients with two of the disorders discussed in this chapter.

Introduction

Purpuric lesions, probably more than any other skin lesion morphology, carry a grave prognosis not shared by most other eruptions. Bleeding or extravasation of red cells into the dermis often results from occlusion and/or destruction of blood vessel walls, both phenomena often resulting from a grave diagnosis. More than most other patients in dermatology, patients who present with purpura undergo extensive systemic evaluation in addition to skin biopsies. Other specialists, such as hematologists and rheumatologists, often participate in the care of these patients; hence, the important value of a dermatology consultation.

The *pathogenetic mechanisms* of purpura may be divided based on different criteria:

1. Systemic (immune complex vasculitis) versus cutaneous (solar purpura)
2. Platelet-related (ITP) versus coagulation abnormalities (proteins C and protein S, anti-phospholipid antibody syndrome)
3. Abnormalities inside the blood vessel (thrombosis) versus in the blood vessel wall (hyalinizing vasculitis) versus the vessel dermal supportive tissue (scurvy)

In the clinical evaluation of purpura, the following determinations are usually valuable:

- Are the lesions inflammatory or not?
- Are they palpable or not?
- Is the eruption diffuse or localized?
- Is the eruption acute or chronic?
- Are the lesions ulcerating or not?

D. F. Mutasim, *Practical Skin Pathology*, DOI 10.1007/978-3-319-14729-1_40

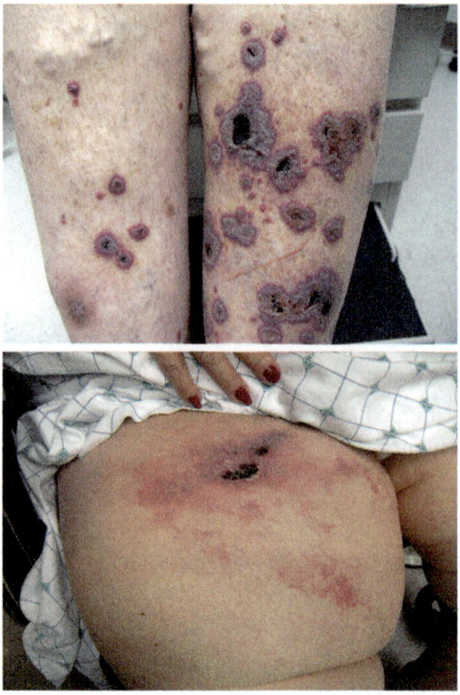

Fig. 40.1 *Upper panel* illustrates a middle-aged man with IgA vasculitis, nephrotic syndrome, and renal failure. Note that some purpuric plaques are centrally ulcerated. *Lower panel* illustrates a middle-aged woman who developed a purpuric and necrotic plaque over the proximal thigh few weeks following initiation of warfarin therapy. Histopathology revealed occlusion of dermal blood vessels by fibrin thrombi characteristic of warfarin necrosis

Inflammatory or Not, and Palpable or Not

Inflammatory purpura is synonymous with vasculitis. In other words, inflammation (erythema and edema) in a purpuric lesion is strong evidence that the patient has vasculitis. A closely related feature to inflammation is palpable infiltration of the lesion. In other words, palpable purpura has been equated to vasculitis and is used by some (usually older dermatologists) as synonymous with vasculitis, in contradistinction to nonpalpable purpura, which is often secondary to a bleeding diathesis or coagulation abnormalities.

When combined together, palpable infiltration and inflammation are almost invariably secondary to vasculitis with the prototype and most common form in the skin being leukocytoclastic vasculitis (LCV), which is also referred to as palpable purpura, immune complex vasculitis, Henoch-Schoeinlin purpura (HSP), and neutrophilic venulitis.

LCV presents acutely, often following an infectious illness or medication, strongly favors the lower legs, is rarely associated with ulcers secondary to skin necrosis, and most often resolves spontaneously. Chronic LCV raises suspicion for an underlying chronic infection, such as hepatitis or autoimmune connective tissue disorder, such as systemic lupus erythematosus and Sjogren syndrome.

Diffuse or Localized

Acute diffuse purpuric eruption is a dermatological emergency. Whether caused by an infection (such as Rocky Mountain spotted fever (RMSF), disseminated meningococcal infection) or disseminated intravascular coagulopathy (DIC; or its closely related disorder, purpura fulminans), a diffuse purpuric eruption carries a grave prognosis and sometimes death.

Localized purpura on the other hand, is secondary either to local physical factors (such as the Valsalva maneuver or a tourniquet), surgical intervention (such as cholesterol emboli, or severing a large vessel in an extremity), or a localized form of DIC, such as in warfarin necrosis.

Acute or Chronic

Acute purpuric eruption is most likely caused by vasculitis or DIC. Chronic purpura, especially in the form of petechiae, is most likely caused by a bleeding diathesis secondary to thrombocytopenia. As mentioned above, vasculitis secondary to an underlying untreated infection (such as chronic hepatitis C) or to an undiagnosed autoimmune connective tissue disorder, may be chronic.

With Ulcers or Without

Purpura associated with ulcers is more often caused by thrombosis rather than vasculitis. This is especially the case with disorders in which a coagulopathy could be identified, such as antiphospholipid antibody syndrome, or drug-induced vasculopathy, such as secondary to cocaine/Levamisole, and in the less-understood disorder, segmental hyalinizing vasculitis (also known as hyalinizing vasculopathy and *atrophie blanche*).

Severe occlusion in LCV may occasionally result in necrosis and ulcer formation; in this setting, a limited number of lesions undergo ulceration.

Unlike patients with antiphospholipid antibody syndrome who present with generally acute to subacute onset ulcers, patients with hyalinizing vasculitis more often present many months after the onset of the lesions. Hyalinizing vasculitis is an insidious disorder in which there is a slowly progressive occlusion of dermal blood vessels followed by ischemic necrosis, purpura, and ulcer formation.

How Helpful Is the Pathology?

Moderately ++

Histological Clues

In the histological evaluation of a biopsy specimen from a purpuric lesion, attention is given to:

- The presence and type of infiltrate
- Whether the pathology is limited to the superficial vascular plexus, or in addition, involves the deeper vascular plexus
- Inflammation of blood vessel walls versus vascular occlusion
- Composition of the occluding material

Type of Infiltrate

Neutrophils

Except for the rare types of granulomatous vasculitis, most cutaneous vasculitis is mediated by neutrophils. Whether the so called lymphocytic vasculitis is a true and primary nosological entity is doubtful. Lymphocytes in lesions of leukemia cutis, lymphoma cutis, and PLEVA may involve blood vessel walls sometimes leading to their destruction. Such histological phenomenon has been referred to sometimes as lymphocytic vasculitis.

Most biopsies from patients with *LCV* reveal easily identifiable histological features. These consist of a superficial neutrophilic infiltrate with nuclear dust in blood vessel walls as well as in their immediate vicinity and in between blood vessel walls, and extravasation of red blood cells. Few eosinophils are often seen and have been suggested to favor medication etiology. Endothelial cells are often swollen, and fibrinous material is deposited in the blood vessel wall, sometimes extending into the lumen resulting in its conclusion.

In the majority of cases, a biopsy specimen that reveals the above features represents allergic or immune complex vasculitis, necessitating a search for an etiology. On a rare occasion, similar findings may be seen in a patient with *infectious vasculitis* where the inciting agent for the vasculitis is not immune complexes, but instead an infectious agent such as the organisms of RMSF, disseminated meningococcemia, Gram negative sepsis, or disseminated fungal infection, including disseminated candidiasis.

Features that raise suspicion for an infectious etiology include involvement of the deep dermal vascular plexus and severe thrombotic occlusion of blood vessels. Fungal organisms may be detected by special stains. Bacterial and rickettsial organisms may be identified by cultures, immunohistochemistry, and PCR. Patients with infectious vasculitis are often sick and hospitalized, except children with chronic meningococcemia.

Lymphocytes

Capillaritis, or pigmented purpuric dermatosis (PPD), is a benign disorder involving papillary dermal capillaries by a lymphocytic infiltrate. Histopathology is often characteristic, and the disorder is generally idiopathic and only rarely secondary to a known agent, such as a medication.

Histiocytes

Granulomatous vasculitis is a small group of disorders that are systemic in nature. Skin lesions are variable. The dermatologist may be asked to evaluate and perform biopsies on patients in order to confirm a suspected diagnosis based on internal organ involvement.

In Wegener's granulomatosis, the upper airways, lung, and kidneys are often affected. The skin lesions may be either similar to those of LCV or to the primary pathology of the disorder, namely necrotizing granulomas. The same is true for Churgg Strauss vasculitis. Lesions may have the characteristic Churgg Strauss granuloma or features of LCV.

The Site of Pathology

As mentioned above, involvement of the deep vascular plexus may raise suspicion for infectious etiology and/or larger blood vessel involvement, raising suspicion for systemic involvement.

Inflammation of Blood Vessel Walls Versus Vascular Occlusion and Composition of the Occluding Material

Infiltration of blood vessel walls by inflammatory cells is synonymous with vasculitis. This is often associated with deposition of fibrin in blood vessel walls, and to a variable degree in the lumen. Deposition of immune complexes on the basement membrane of blood vessel walls activates the complement system and attracts neutrophils, which damage the vessel wall thus activating the coagulation pathway. Fibrinogen is transformed to fibrin in the latter stages of coagulation.

The histopathology of purpura secondary to *primary occlusive disorders* resides primarily in the lumen, and the occlusive material varies depending on the underlying cause.

In the various coagulopathies, whether due to antiphospholipid antibodies, coagulation factor abnormalities, mixed cryoglobulinemia, or DIC, the occluding material is fibrin, a reddish granular and/or fibrillar material. In monoclonal cryoglobulinemia, the material is cryoglobulin, which appears more homogeneous. In disorders of platelets, such as heparin-induced thrombocytopenia, occlusion is with platelet-rich thrombi. In thromboembolic phenomena (including cholesterol emboli), the occlusion is with atheromatous material, often containing cholesterol clefts.

Finally, in the less well understood disorder known as a *hyalinizing vasculopathy*, segmental hyalinizing vasculitis and *atrophie blanche*, it is believed that the vascular occlusion results from defects in fibrinolysis, that is, the predisposition is not for excessive deposition of fibrin but instead of deficiency in the normal mechanisms of fibrin lysis.

Conclusions

In the evaluation of a patient with purpuric lesions, several questions need to be addressed, some clinical, others histological, and yet others hematological and systemic.

Chapter 41
Blisters

Figure 41.1 illustrates four patients with four of the disorders discussed in this chapter.

Introduction

Many skin disorders may have blisters. In some, the blisters are secondary and occur occasionally or rarely. Examples include lichen planus (LP) and erythema multiforme (EM). These disorders are generally nonblistering; but in a few patients, some of the lesions may develop blisters due to severe degeneration of the basal layer. These disorders will not be discussed here as each disorder usually retains its characteristic features in other lesions, so clinical recognition is generally easy.

Some common infections result in blisters. These include viruses, such as herpes simplex virus, varicella-zoster virus, and Coxsackie virus; bacteria, such as *Staphylococcus aureus*, superficial fungi, and *Candida*. The clinical characteristics in these disorders usually suffice to make an accurate clinical diagnosis. In some cases, cultures may be indicated. These disorders will also not be discussed.

Sometimes blisters arise due to epidermal necrosis. This occurs in many skin disorders whose primary clinical presentation is sloughing. These include physical factors, such as severe sunburn, extreme heat or extreme cold, and acute radiation; chemical factors, such as exposure to acid or alkali; and reaction to medication, such as Steven–Johnson Syndrome (SJS) and toxic epidermal necrolysis (TEN). Again, these disorders will not be discussed here (discussed in Chap. 33).

Instead, this section addresses disorders that reveal blisters as the primary lesion and are referred to as primary bullous disorders. Many are autoimmune in pathogenesis.

D. F. Mutasim, *Practical Skin Pathology*, DOI 10.1007/978-3-319-14729-1_41

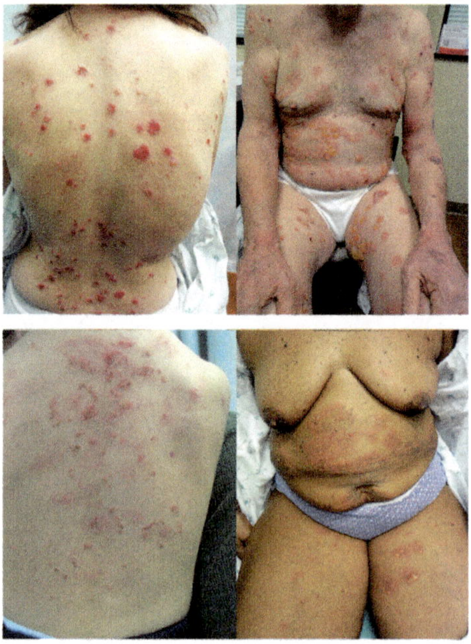

Fig. 41.1 *Left upper panel* shows a middle-aged woman with generalized painful erosions of pemphigus vulgaris. *Right upper panel* shows an old man with generalized bullous pemphigoid. *Right lower panel* shows an older woman with inflammatory epidermolysis bullosa acquisita. Note the similarity of lesions to bullous pemphigoid. *Left lower panel* shows a 10-year-old boy with pemphigus herpetiformis. Note shallow erosions. Multiple biopsies showed eosinophilic spongiosis and immunofluorescence showed IgG around epidermal cells

Classification

There is more than one approach to the diagnosis of a bullous disorder. The following approach takes into consideration distribution of lesions, predominant morphology, and possible inducing factors.

I. Generalized predominantly intact blisters
   BP, EBA, LAD, DH, SLE
II. Generalized, with extensive erosions
   PV, PF, PNP
III. Limited to the legs
   Edema, diabetes mellitus (DM), pretibial epidermolysis bullosa (EB), localized bullous pemphigoid (BP)
IV. Localized trauma-induced
   PCT, pseudo-PCT, EBA

Generalized with Predominantly Intact Blisters

BP, EBA, LAD, DH, SLE

Clinical Clues

This group consists of five autoimmune disorders, all of which are subepidermal (BP, epidermolysis bullosa acquisita (EBA II), linear IgA disease (LAD), dermatitis herpetiformis (DH), and the bullous eruption of systemic lupus erythematosus (SLE)).

Some clinical features may favor one disorder over the others. For example, predominant involvement over the joints and extensor surfaces, especially if lesions are small, strongly favors DH. In at least two-thirds of the patients with BP, lesions strongly favor skin folds, especially the inner thighs. EBA II mimics BP strongly; unlike EBA type I in which lesions are generally trauma induced and frequently heal with milia, lesions in EBA II are surrounded by inflammation, just as in BP.

LAD may also mimic BP to a large degree except in hospitalized patients, where it presents more acutely and secondary to a drug, such as vancomycin. The bullous eruption of SLE occurs in patients usually known to have SLE. Lesions are often scattered randomly without favoring photodistributed areas or having a characteristic pattern. Many blisters often arise within urticarial plaques. Except for classic DH and classic BP, histological and immunofluorescence examination is absolutely necessary.

Histological Clues

The ideal specimen for histological evaluation of a blistering eruption is a shave biopsy specimen that includes a vesicle with surrounding intact skin. The border of the vesicle often reveals the earliest changes that result in blistering, and that are important in making a diagnosis.

All the above disorders reveal a subepidermal blister with an underlying superficial dermal infiltrate that may also be seen in the overlying epidermis and in the blister cavity. The infiltrate is predominantly or exclusively neutrophilic in all except BP, in which the infiltrate is predominantly or exclusively eosinophilic. In general, neutrophil-predominant infiltrates in the skin tend to contain some eosinophils and eosinophil predominant infiltrates tend to contain some neutrophils.

A patient with BP may have only urticarial pre-bullous lesions, so-called urticarial pemphigoid. Histology often reveals eosinophilic spongiosis and/or an eosinophilic infiltrate along the dermal–epidermal junction.

Immunofluorescence

The diagnosis of an autoimmune bullous disorder is based on its antibody specificity, that is, the protein or antigen in the skin that the patient's antibodies are directed against. This can be obtained by ELISA using the patient's serum and a source of antigen. This test, however, is not commercially widely available yet. Immunofluorescence is a powerful substitute.

Direct immunofluorescence is performed on noninflamed and nonblistered skin immediately adjacent to a blister or inflamed skin. The biopsy specimen is placed in a special medium (ammonium sulfate) that does not permanently fix and disrupt the structure of proteins, allowing their detection by binding to antibodies, which are labeled with fluorescent material that makes them visible under a fluorescence microscope.

IgG deposition along the basement membrane is characteristic of BP, EBA, and the bullous eruption of SLE; while IgA deposition is characteristic of DH and LAD.

IgA deposition in DH is characteristically granular along the basement membrane and strongly favors the tips of dermal papillae over the shoulders and tips of the rete, a pattern that mimics the distribution of neutrophils histologically. LAD is characterized by continuous linear deposition of IgA along the dermal epidermal junction. While C3 deposition is seen in almost all cases of DH, C3 is present in approximately 50 % of the cases of LAD.

In BP, deposition of C3 and IgG is present in all cases. IgG is generally less intense than C3. In EBA, however, deposition of IgG and C3 tends to be either equal in intensity or IgG of higher intensity than C3. Differentiation between BP and EBA based solely on direct immunofluorescence is not possible. In order to differentiate between BP and EBA with certainty, a slightly more complex immunofluorescence test may be performed.

The *salt split immunofluorescence* technique consists of taking the submitted biopsy specimen out of the frozen state, thawing it and incubating it with a solution of sodium chloride, which results in a subepidermal split within several hours to 2 days. The new specimen is subjected to direct immunofluorescence.

In EBA, the whole deposition (IgG and C3) is limited to the dermal side with no deposition over the epidermal side. In BP, deposition of IgG and C3 is either limited to the epidermal side only or divided between the epidermal and dermal side.

Sometimes the submitted specimen contains a blister so the salt split technique cannot be performed. In this case, a somewhat similar procedure may be performed but instead on the serum of the patient and normal human skin that has been incubated with sodium chloride. The antibodies in the serum of patients with EBA bind to the dermal side only while antibodies from the serum of patients with BP bind either the epidermal side or both epidermal and dermal side.

Direct immunofluorescence in the bullous eruption of SLE is similar to EBA and the two disorders can be distinguished based on the presence or not of SLE. That is why some authors suggest that the bullous eruption of SLE is a type of EBA. In this analysis, patients with SLE are viewed to make several autoantibodies, among them antibodies to collagen VII, the EBA antigen, which then cause blisters akin to EBA.

Generalized with Extensive Erosions

Clinical Clues

Unlike the above group of subepidermal bullous disorders, the blisters in this group are secondary to intraepidermal acantholysis. The disorders are pemphigus vulgaris (PV), pemphigus foliaceous (PF), and paraneoplastic pemphigus (PNP). Although the primary lesion in these disorders is a blister, the lesions are flaccid and rupture easily, resulting in erosions. Often, patients may present predominantly or solely with erosions. Unlike the above group of disorders in which erosions may heal spontaneously, erosions in pemphigus tend to persist, and advance if not treated.

The average duration of disease from onset until diagnosis of PV is 13 months. This is due to the fact that in the vast majority of patients, the initial lesions are mucosal (almost universally oral) and may be missed for other oral erosive disorders, especially if patients are initially evaluated by physicians who are not dermatologists or who do not have experience in pemphigus. PNP is generally an acute disorder with involvement of multiple mucous membranes and the skin. Lesions are polymorphous, mimicking PV, BP, LP, EM, and SJS. Most patients have known underlying neoplasms, especially of the hematopoietic system (specifically B-cell neoplasms).

Histological Clues

PV is characterized by suprabasal acantolysis without dyskeratosis, making differentiation from other acantholytic disorders easy. Similarly, PF reveals superficial intraepidermal acantholysis (within the granular layer or in between the granular and the horny layers) and should be differentiated from bullous impetigo (neutrophils in the blister cavity) and Staphylococcal scalded skin syndrome (SSSS) (which cannot be differentiated histologically, but by immunofluorescence). Variants of PF (pemphigus erythematosus, drug-induced pemphigus) have similar histopathology, except pemphigus herpetiformis, which is characterized by eosinophilic spongiosis without obvious acantholysis.

PNP has a polymorphous histological presentation just as it does clinically. Some cases are identical histologically to PV, while others mimic EM, and yet others may show features of both PV and EM in the same lesion. A strong index of suspicion is usually required to consider the diagnosis. In the absence of acantholysis, a drug eruption may be histologically suspected, as patients with PNP often are taking many medications.

Immunofluorescence

Direct immunofluorescence in all three types of pemphigus reveals deposition of IgG around epidermal cells. The deposition may favor the lower epidermal cell layers in PV and the outer layers in PF, but not consistently. C3 is also frequently deposited in a similar pattern, but is of little diagnostic value. IgG deposition is required regardless of the presence and intensity of C3 in order to make the diagnosis.

In addition to the intraepidermal deposition of IgG, PNP often reveals deposition of C3 along the basement membrane, but with lesser intensity and continuity than that in BP.

Indirect immunofluorescence in all three pemphigus types reveals antibodies in the patients' sera against adhesion molecules on the surface of stratified squamous epithelial cells. The most sensitive substrate is monkey esophagus. PNP antibodies bind multiple other tissues and organs, including simple and transitional epithelium, such as the gastrointestinal tract and urinary ladder. Rat bladder is approximately 80 % sensitive and specific for the detection of PNP antibodies compared with PV and PF.

Blisters Limited to the Legs

Clinical Clues

Edema blisters, diabetic bulla, localized BP, and pretibial EB all favor the lower legs.

Edema blisters occur in the setting of severe leg edema usually of acute rather than chronic nature, often in hospitalized patients, are usually several centimeters large, and lack evidence of surrounding inflammation. Unlike edema blisters, *diabetic blisters* tend to wax and wane, and occur with no apparent precipitating factors. While edema blisters result from severe accumulation of fluid in the superficial dermis, diabetic blisters result from dissolution of a weak basement membrane believed to be due to excessive glycosylation of basement membrane proteins.

Localized BP was initially reported to occur in the head and neck area (known as Brunsting-Perry pemphigoid) but was soon recognized to also occur on the lower leg and occasionally elsewhere. Lesions may initially occur on one leg but often become bilateral. They are similar in appearance to lesions of generalized BP. In some cases, only the feet are involved. The diagnosis is often missed for severe allergic contact dermatitis, stasis dermatitis, and bullous tinea. In the author's experience, the diagnosis is often delayed by several months. Rarely does the disorder become generalized, usually after few years. The author has seen only two such patients among approximately 12 patients with leg BP.

The diagnosis of *Pretibial EB* is often delayed by several years. Unlike other types of EB in which the onset is in the newborn or infancy periods, the onset of pretibial EB is in adulthood. Although the disorder is autosomal dominantly inherited, in the author's experience of three cases, no positive family history could be elicited. Lesions are often associated with scarring and milia. The subepidermal vesicles in this disorder are accompanied by a superficial lymphocytic infiltrate; hence, they are often misdiagnosed histologically for an inflammatory disorder and treated with topical steroids. A strong index of suspicion and negative direct immunofluorescence are necessary to make the diagnosis of this rare disorder.

Histological Clues

Histological findings are at least moderately helpful among the four disorders. Severe edema is usually obvious in biopsy specimens of edema blisters. No epidermal pathology or dermal infiltrate is seen. Diabetic blisters are also subepidermal and lack inflammation, and may be mistaken for noninflammatory EBA (EBA I) and porphyria cutanea tarda (PCT). Histological findings in localized BP are similar to those in generalized BP, namely, a subepidermal vesicle with eosinophils. Pretibial EB is characterized by a subepidermal blister with usually dense superficial lymphocytic infiltrate, and scar fibrosis (this disorder is among the dystrophic types of EB). The presence of scarring clinically or histologically is a major clue to the diagnosis in a patient with chronic trauma-induced blisters of the shins. Due of the extreme rarity of the disorder, it is rarely suspected histologically. In the three cases that I have seen, biopsy reports have carried diagnoses, such as bullous lichen planus, lichen sclerosis, EBA, and scar, with overlying subepidermal vesicle.

Immunofluorescence

Direct immunofluorescence is negative in the above disorders except localized BP in which it is similar to generalized BP.

Localized Trauma-Induced Blisters

Blisters in PCT, pseudo-PCT, and EBA I (also called mechanobullous type) all result from trauma, including friction. In EBA, basement membrane destruction and easy blistering result from binding of EBA antibodies to type VII collagen in the sublamina densa region of the basement membrane. In PCT, the phototoxic reaction caused by high skin levels of porphyrin occurs predominantly in chronically sun-exposed skin. This results in skin fragility, leading to blistering or sloughing-off easily as a result of minor trauma.

All three disorders are characterized by a noninflammatory subepidermal vesicle. Superficial scar fibrosis and thickening of superficial blood vessel walls may be seen in chronically affected skin.

Direct immunofluorescence reveals deposition of IgG and C3 along the basement membrane in EBA, while PCT and pseudo-PCT are characterized by generally moderate deposition of IgG and IgA and, to a lesser degree, other immune deposits in superficial blood vessel walls and less frequently the basement membrane. Pseudo-PCT may be differentiated from PCT by the lack of elevated urinary porphyrins and the easily provided history of excessive ultraviolet exposure along with the intake of a phototoxic medication.

Conclusions

In approaching the diagnosis of a patient with blisters, a combination of history, physical findings, histopathology, and direct immunofluorescence results in an accurate diagnosis in the vast majority of patients. Indirect immunofluorescence is required only rarely.

Index

D. F. Mutasim, *Practical Skin Pathology*, DOI 10.1007/978-3-319-14729-1

Printed by Printforce, the Netherlands